MW00875090

DR. SARA J. CAMERON, PhD

The Warrior Within

Triumphing Over Cancer with the Mind

ËL PUBLICATIONS   PENNSYLVANIA

Copyright © [2021] by Sara Cameron

All rights reserved.

This work is owned by Ël Publications and is protected by copyright laws. Without the written consent of the copyright holder, it cannot be duplicated, copied, or disseminated in any way. This work's unauthorized use or dissemination is punishable by both civil and criminal laws.

Condition of Sales

This book is sold subject to the condition that it shall not, by way of trade or otherwise, be lent, resold, hired out or otherwise circulated without the publishers prior consent in any form of binding on cover other than that in which it is published and without a similar condition, including this condition being imposed on the subsequent purchaser.

TABLE OF CONTENTS

AUTHOR'S NOTE

Dearest Warrior,

Welcome to a transformative exploration of the remarkable power that resides within each and every one of us—the power of the mind. In this book, we embark on a journey that unveils the untapped potential within, where the mind becomes an extraordinary catalyst for healing, resilience, and personal transformation.

Over a decade and half of working as a specialist, I was inspired by the countless stories of individuals who defied the odds, transcended their circumstances, and experienced extraordinary healing through the power of their thoughts, emotions, and beliefs. It is their remarkable stories which inspired me to share with you what you are about to delve into in the following pages.

This is not a book about dismissing or replacing medical treatment. Rather, it is an exploration of the dynamic interplay between our minds and our bodies, shining a light on the profound impact our thoughts and emotions have on our physical well-being. It is a testament to the inherent capacity we possess to participate actively in our own healing process.

In these chapters, we will journey through the intricate pathways of the mind-body connection. We will uncover the influence of stress, emotions, and belief systems on our health, and we will witness the awe-inspiring ways in which our mental outlook can shape our healing trajectory. We also aim at exploring the field of psychoneuroimmunology, revealing the intimate relationship between our thoughts, emotions, and immune system.

Throughout this book, we will explore practical strategies and techniques to harness the power of our minds in the face of cancer. From mindfulness practices that cultivate resilience to visualization exercises that tap into the mind's potential for healing, you will discover a wealth of tools to empower and support your journey.

I want to extend my deepest gratitude to the brave individuals who shared their personal stories and insights, as well as the dedicated healthcare professionals and researchers who continue to expand our understanding of the mind's role in healing. It is their collective wisdom that infuses these pages with hope, inspiration, and a renewed sense of possibility.

As you embark on this transformative journey, I invite you to approach these pages with an open heart and an open mind. Embrace the power of curiosity, as it will guide you through the depths of understanding and self-discovery. Remember, this is not a journey to be rushed; it is an invitation to immerse yourself in the exploration of your own innate potential for healing and transformation.

May this book serve as a guiding light, illuminating the path towards a mind-body connection that empowers you in your healing journey. May it remind you of your inner strength and resilience, and may it ignite a spark of hope that propels you forward, even in the face of adversity.

Thank you for embarking on this transformative journey with me. Together, let us discover the extraordinary power of the mind and unlock the infinite possibilities that await us.

With deepest gratitude and warmest wishes,

Sarah J. Cameron

INTRODUCTION

Gaining Deeper Understanding

THE POWER OF THE MIND IN THE CANCER RECOVERY JOURNEY

In the depths of a cancer diagnosis, the journey towards healing can often seem arduous and uncertain. It is a time when physical strength is tested, emotions run deep, and the soul searches for solace. It is during these challenging moments that the extraordinary power of the mind emerges, offering a beacon of hope and a pathway to transformation.

This book explores the awe-inspiring healing potential of the mind in the cancer recovery journey. It delves into the depths of the human spirit, where the mind holds the key to unlocking inner strength, resilience, and a renewed sense of purpose. With a blend of professional expertise and heartfelt compassion, we invite you on a journey that illuminates the immense power residing within you.

Scientific research has increasingly recognized the profound impact of the mind on the body's ability to heal. Our thoughts, emotions, and beliefs influence our physiological responses, shaping the trajectory of our recovery.

In the early 1800s, there existed a peculiar case that shed light on the extraordinary power of the mind in influencing one's physical health. This story revolves around a man named Émile Coué, a pharmacist who inadvertently became a pioneer in the field of mind-body medicine.

Émile Coué was not a typical medical professional. He possessed an unwavering belief in the innate healing power of the mind. He observed that many of his patients who received treatment with the same medications exhibited varying levels of improvement. This led him to ponder the role of the mind in healing and to develop a groundbreaking concept known as "auto-suggestion."

One particular incident left a profound impact on Coué's understanding of the mind's influence on health. He encountered a patient who suffered from a severe case of paralysis. This individual was convinced that he would never regain control of his legs. Coué recognized the man's psychological state as a major obstacle to his recovery. Determined to prove the power of the mind, Coué approached the patient and gently suggested that he was getting better with each passing day.

To his astonishment, the patient experienced a gradual improvement in his condition. He regained movement in his legs, and his paralysis subsided. This remarkable transformation ignited Coué's curiosity and set him on a path to explore the potential of the mind in healing.

The story of Émile Coué and his patients serves as a testament to the profound impact of psychological factors on physical health. It highlights the immense power of the mind in influencing our well-being and the potential for self-directed healing. While this story may be an extreme example, it underscores the importance of cultivating a positive mindset, embracing hope, and harnessing the power of belief.

But the power of the mind in the cancer recovery journey goes beyond physical healing. It holds the key to igniting a profound inner transformation, where individuals discover a renewed sense of purpose and meaning. Cancer is a formidable adversary, challenging us to confront our fears, reassess our priorities, and delve deep into the recesses of our souls. It serves as a catalyst for personal growth and invites us to rediscover what truly matters in life.

Through the power of the mind, individuals embark on a journey of self-discovery, guided by introspection, self-compassion, and a reawakening of their inner desires and aspirations. It is in this process that renewed purpose emerges, infusing each moment with a newfound sense of meaning and joy. The cancer recovery journey becomes an opportunity for profound transformation, where individuals emerge not only as survivors but as thrivers, embracing life with a depth and authenticity they may have never known before.

In the pages of this book, we will explore the multifaceted dimensions of the mind's power in the cancer recovery journey. We will delve into practical techniques and strategies to cultivate a positive mindset, nurture emotional well-being, and foster innser strength. Drawing from the experiences of individuals who have triumphed over cancer, we will share stories of resilience, inspiration, and profound transformation.

1

UNVEILING THE ENIGMA OF CANCER: EXPLORING THE DEPTHS OF A COMPLEX DISEASE

In the medical world, there is perhaps no word more feared, more laden with uncertainty, than cancer. It is an adversary that strikes without warning, disrupting lives and shattering dreams. But amidst the shadows of despair, there exists a flicker of hope—a beacon of strength that illuminates the path towards understanding and resilience. This chapter marks the beginning of our exploration as we embark on a captivating journey to unravel the enigma of cancer, unraveling its mysteries while empowering you with knowledge, compassion, and the unwavering belief in the power of healing.

Cancer, a word etched into the depths of our collective consciousness, is an intricate dance of cells gone awry. Within the vast tapestry of the human body, trillions of cells harmoniously coexist, dividing and multiplying with precision. But in the face of cancer, this intricate symphony is disrupted—a rogue cell rebels against the natural order, multiplying uncontrollably, and refusing to succumb to the body's regulatory mechanisms.

At its core, cancer is a complex and heterogeneous disease characterized by the uncontrolled growth and spread of abnormal cells. These renegade cells form a mass called a tumor, which can invade nearby tissues and organs, impairing their normal functions. If left unchecked, cancerous cells can also break away from the primary tumor and travel through the bloodstream or lymphatic system to establish new colonies in distant parts of the body—an ominous process known as metastasis.

HOW CANCER OPERATES

To comprehend the intricacies of cancer, we must journey into the microscopic realm of cells, where the battle between health and disease unfolds. Like a detective on the trail of a hidden truth, we delve into the origins of cancer, striving to understand its causes.

Let us embark on precisely that expedition, aiming to demystify the intricate mechanisms that drive this formidable adversary. Prepare yourself to be captivated and enlightened as we delve into the world of cancer, unraveling its operations in a manner that is accessible to all, irrespective of prior medical knowledge.

THE CELLULAR BATTLEFIELD: UNDERSTANDING THE BASICS

At the heart of the battle between health and cancer lies a microscopic arena—the human cell. To comprehend how cancer operates, we must first grasp the fundamental principles of cellular biology. Picture cells as the building blocks of life, each with its own specific role and function within the body. In a healthy state, cells replicate and divide in a controlled manner, ensuring the proper growth, maintenance, and repair of tissues and organs.

Now, imagine a rebellion within this harmonious community of cells—a group of cells that breaks free from the constraints of regulation. These cells, known as cancer cells, are the seeds from which cancer originates. But how do these rebels emerge, and what drives their insubordination?

Cancer often arises due to genetic alterations within cells. These alterations, or mutations, can be inherited from our parents or acquired during our lifetime due to various factors such as exposure to carcinogens or spontaneous errors in DNA replication. These mutations disrupt the delicate balance of cell division and death, leading to uncontrolled cell growth and the formation of tumors.

As the rebellious cells continue to proliferate, they clump together, forming a mass called a tumor. Tumors can be classified into two main types: benign and malignant. Benign tumors are relatively harmless, confined to a specific area and unlikely to spread to other parts of the body. Malignant tumors, on the other hand, are the true culprits of cancer— they have the ability to invade nearby tissues and spread to distant sites through a process known as metastasis.

Metastasis is a menacing aspect of cancer, allowing it to infiltrate different parts of the body and establish secondary colonies. Picture cancer cells as cunning infiltrators, employing various strategies to invade new territories. They can enter the bloodstream or lymphatic system, hitching a ride to distant organs, where they can proliferate and wreak havoc. The ability of cancer to metastasize significantly affects its prognosis and treatment options.

As cancer cells multiply and establish themselves, they require a robust blood supply to sustain their growth. This is where angiogenesis, the process of forming new blood vessels, comes into play. Cancer cells release signals that stimulate nearby blood vessels to sprout and provide them with the necessary nutrients and oxygen. The formation of an extensive network of blood vessels within a tumor ensures its survival and enables its aggressive expansion.

The human body possesses an intricate defense system—the immune system—that detects and eliminates abnormal cells, including cancer cells. However, cancer has evolved ingenious strategies to evade the immune system's surveillance and destruction. It can disguise itself, camouflage its antigens, and inhibit the immune response, effectively outsmarting the body's natural defenses.

Also, cancer cells are not isolated entities; they exist within a complex environment known as the tumor microenvironment. This environment comprises a diverse array of cells, including immune cells, fibroblasts, and blood vessels. Through paracrine signaling, cancer cells communicate with neighboring cells, influencing their behavior and co-opting them to support tumor growth and progression. This communication network plays a critical role in fostering a favorable environment for cancer cells and facilitating their invasion into surrounding tissues.

Cancer cells are notorious for their genetic instability—a characteristic that fuels their adaptability and resistance to treatment. Genetic instability refers to the high rate of genetic mutations and alterations within cancer cells, resulting in a diverse population of cells with varying genetic profiles. This diversity enables cancer cells to acquire advantageous traits, such as drug resistance or the ability to evade therapies. Understanding genetic instability is vital for developing targeted treatments that can effectively combat the ever-changing landscape of cancer cells.

Cancer knows no boundaries as it can emerge in any organ, tissue, or system within the body. This is why there is a rich tapestry of cancer's diversity. Ranging from breast cancer, lung cancer, prostate cancer, colorectal cancer—the list extends to encompass numerous forms, each with its unique characteristics and challenges.

Carcinomas, originating from epithelial tissues, are the most common type of cancer, accounting for about 80% to 90% of all cases. They can arise in various organs such as the breast, lung, colon, prostate, and skin. Sarcomas, on the other hand, arise from connective tissues such as bone, muscle, and cartilage. Lymphomas and leukemias affect the blood-forming cells and the lymphatic system, respectively. Central nervous system cancers, including brain tumors, originate in the brain and spinal cord. These are just a few examples of the vast array of cancers that exist.

We have gotten a glimpse of the manner of the relentless progression of this horrendous disease. Armed with this newfound knowledge, we can confront cancer with determination and understanding.

TYPES OF CANCER

To comprehend the various types of cancer, it is also essential to grasp the cellular intricacies that underlie each firm of the disease, the various modes of operation as well as the symptoms.

BREAST CANCER: A GENDER-SPECIFIC BATTLE

Breast cancer originates when these abnormal cells begin to multiply within the breast tissue. It can occur in both men and women, although it is more common in women. The precise causes of breast cancer remain complex and multifaceted, often involving a combination of genetic and environmental factors.

Two primary types of breast cancer exist; *ductal carcinoma* and *lobular carcinoma*. Ductal carcinoma originates in the milk ducts, which act as the pathways for milk to reach the nipple. Lobular carcinoma, on the other hand, originates in the lobules, which produce milk. These two types may further branch out into various subtypes, each possessing unique characteristics and treatment approaches.

THE DOMINO EFFECT

Similar to other forms of cancer, breast cancer's true menace lies in its ability to spread to other parts of the body. This process, known as metastasis, occurs when cancer cells break away from the primary tumor and travel through the bloodstream or lymphatic system to distant organs, such as the bones, lungs, liver, or brain. This metastatic spread transforms breast cancer into a systemic disease, demanding comprehensive treatment strategies.

IDENTIFYING THE WARNING SIGNS

Understanding the signs and symptoms of breast cancer is vital for early detection. While some individuals may experience no noticeable symptoms, others may observe the following indicators:

1. The growth of a lump or thickening in the breast or underarm area.
2. Changes in breast size or shape.
3. Dimpling or puckering of the skin on the breast.
4. Nipple discharge or inversion.
5. Redness or swelling of the breast or nipple.
6. Persistent breast or nipple pain.

Remember, these symptoms are not exclusive to breast cancer and can be caused by various factors. It is crucial to consult a healthcare professional for an accurate diagnosis.

SCREENING AND DIAGNOSIS

Screening plays a vital role in detecting breast cancer at its earliest stages. Mammography, a low-dose X-ray of the breast, is the gold standard for breast cancer screening. Additional imaging techniques such as ultrasound or magnetic resonance imaging (MRI) may be employed when necessary.

If an abnormality is detected during screening or if symptoms are present, a biopsy is performed. During this procedure, a small tissue sample is extracted from the suspicious area and examined under a microscope by a pathologist. This analysis confirms the presence of cancer and provides essential information about its type, grade, and hormone receptor status.

PROSTATE CANCER: A MALE-SPECIFIC CONCERN

Prostate cancer originates when these abnormal cells begin to multiply within the prostate gland, a small walnut-shaped organ located beneath the bladder and in front of the rectum. The prostate gland is responsible for producing seminal fluid, which nourishes and transports sperm. Prostate cancer is predominantly a disease that affects men.

The exact causes of prostate cancer remain intricate and multifactorial, often involving a combination of genetic and environmental factors. Age also plays a significant role, as the risk of developing prostate cancer increases with advancing years.

IDENTIFYING THE WARNING SIGNS

Detecting prostate cancer in its early stages is crucial for effective treatment. While prostate cancer may not cause noticeable symptoms in its early stages, there are certain indicators that warrant attention:

1.   *Urinary Changes.* Frequent urination, especially at night, weak urine flow, difficulty starting or stopping urination, or a feeling of incomplete bladder emptying.
2.   *Blood in Urine or Semen.* Unexplained blood in urine or semen may be a sign of prostate cancer.
3.   *Erectile Dysfunction.* Difficulty achieving or maintaining an erection may be linked to prostate cancer.

4. *Pelvic Discomfort.* Pain or discomfort in the pelvic area, hips, lower back, or upper thighs can be associated with advanced prostate cancer.

While examining these symptoms, it is also necessary to remember that these symptoms can also be caused by conditions other than prostate cancer. Consultation with a healthcare professional is crucial for accurate diagnosis.

SCREENING AND DIAGNOSIS

Screening serves as a valuable tool in detecting prostate cancer at an early stage. The most common screening method is the prostate-specific antigen (PSA) blood test. Elevated levels of PSA can indicate the presence of prostate cancer or other prostate-related conditions. Additional tests, such as a digital rectal examination (DRE) or imaging studies, may be recommended based on the initial screening results.

To confirm a diagnosis of prostate cancer, a biopsy is typically performed. During this procedure, small tissue samples are extracted from the prostate gland and examined under a microscope by a pathologist. The biopsy provides crucial information about the cancer's aggressiveness, enabling healthcare professionals to develop an appropriate treatment plan.

LUNG CANCER: CONFRONTING THE IMPACTS OF TOBACCO

Lung cancer originates when these abnormal cells begin to multiply within the lungs. The lungs, crucial organs for respiration, are responsible for inhaling oxygen and exhaling carbon dioxide. Lung cancer primarily affects individuals who have a history of smoking, although non-smokers can also develop this disease due to other factors such as exposure to secondhand smoke, environmental pollutants, or genetic predisposition.

IDENTIFYING THE WARNING SIGNS

Detecting lung cancer in its early stages can significantly impact treatment outcomes. While symptoms may not be apparent in the early stages, certain indicators should not be ignored:

1. *Persistent Cough.* A persistent or worsening cough that lasts for more than a few weeks, particularly if accompanied by coughing up blood or rust-colored sputum.
2. *Shortness of Breath.* Breathlessness or wheezing, which may occur during physical activity or even at rest.
3. *Chest Pain.* Dull, aching chest pain that may worsen with deep breathing, laughing, or coughing.
4. *Unexplained Weight Loss.* Sudden and unexplained weight loss, accompanied by loss of appetite and fatigue.
5. *Recurring Respiratory Infections.* Frequent respiratory infections, such as bronchitis or pneumonia, that do not respond to usual treatments.

If you experience any of these warning signs, consult a healthcare professional for a proper evaluation.

SCREENING AND DIAGNOSIS

Screening plays a crucial role in the early detection of lung cancer, especially for individuals at high risk, such as current or former smokers. Low-dose computed tomography (CT) scans are commonly used for lung cancer screening. These scans can detect small abnormalities in the lungs that may indicate the presence of cancer.

To confirm a diagnosis of lung cancer, further tests are necessary. These may include additional imaging studies, such as positron emission tomography (PET) scans, and a biopsy. During a biopsy, a small sample of lung tissue is obtained, either through a needle or during a surgical procedure, and examined under a microscope by a pathologist. This analysis helps determine the type and stage of the cancer, guiding the appropriate treatment approach.

COLORECTAL CANCER: JOURNEYING THROUGH THE DIGESTIVE TRACT

Colorectal cancer originates when these abnormal cells begin to multiply within the lining of the colon or rectum. The colon and rectum, crucial parts of the digestive system, play a vital role in processing food, absorbing nutrients, and eliminating waste. Colorectal cancer is one of the most common cancers worldwide and typically affects individuals over the age of 50, although it can occur in younger individuals as well.

IDENTIFYING THE WARNING SIGNS

Detecting colorectal cancer at its earliest stages is crucial for successful treatment outcomes. While symptoms may not be evident in the early stages, certain indicators should not be ignored:

1. *Changes in Bowel Habits.* Persistent changes in bowel habits, such as diarrhea, constipation, or a change in stool consistency, lasting more than a few weeks.

2. *Rectal Bleeding.* Blood in the stool, either bright red or dark, tarry stools, may indicate colorectal cancer.

3. *Abdominal Discomfort.* Persistent abdominal pain, cramping, or discomfort, particularly when accompanied by bloating or gas.

4. *Unexplained Weight Loss.* Sudden and unexplained weight loss, accompanied by a loss of appetite and fatigue.

5. *Fatigue and Weakness.* Persistent fatigue, weakness, or a general feeling of being unwell, which may be indicative of anemia.

Still on a cautionary note, these symptoms can also be caused by conditions other than colorectal cancer. If you experience any of these warning signs, it is advisable to consult a healthcare professional for a proper evaluation.

SCREENING AND DIAGNOSIS

Screening plays a pivotal role in the early detection of colorectal cancer, even in the absence of symptoms. Several screening methods are available, including stool-based tests, such as the fecal occult blood test (FOBT) or fecal immunochemical test (FIT), which detect hidden blood in the stool. Additionally, colonoscopy, a procedure that allows visualization of the colon and rectum, can both detect and remove precancerous growths called polyps.

If an abnormality is detected during screening or if symptoms are present, further diagnostic tests may be performed. These may include imaging studies, such as a CT scan or magnetic resonance imaging (MRI), and a biopsy. During a biopsy, a small sample of tissue is extracted from the colon or rectum and examined under a microscope by a pathologist. This analysis confirms the presence of cancer and provides essential information about its type, stage, and aggressiveness.

SKIN CANCER: THE VISIBLE CONSEQUENCES OF SUN EXPOSURE

Skin cancer emerges when certain cells in the skin undergo abnormal changes, leading to uncontrolled growth and the formation of tumors. The three main types of skin cancer are basal cell carcinoma, squamous cell carcinoma, and melanoma. Each type originates from different cells within the skin and exhibits distinct characteristics and potential for spreading.

IDENTIFYING THE WARNING SIGNS

Early detection of skin cancer is crucial for successful treatment outcomes. Regular self-examinations and awareness of warning signs are paramount. Common indicators of skin cancer include:

1. *Changes in Moles or Lesions.* Pay attention to moles or skin lesions that change in size, shape, color, or texture over time.
2. *New Growths.* Be mindful of the appearance of new growths on the skin, especially those that are irregular, asymmetrical, or have uneven borders.
3. *Sores that Do Not Heal.* Persistent sores that fail to heal, or wounds that re-open, may warrant further evaluation.

4. *Bleeding or Oozing.* Moles or lesions that bleed, itch, or ooze may indicate the presence of skin cancer.

5. *Itching or Sensitivity.* Skin areas that become itchy, tender, or overly sensitive should be examined by a healthcare professional.

If you notice any of these warning signs, it is essential to consult a healthcare professional promptly for a thorough evaluation.

DIAGNOSIS AND TREATMENT

Diagnosing skin cancer involves a comprehensive assessment of the affected area and may require a biopsy, where a small sample of tissue is taken for examination. Once a diagnosis is confirmed, the treatment plan is tailored to the type, stage, and location of the cancer, as well as the patient's overall health.

LEUKEMIA: THE INTRICATE BATTLE WITHIN THE BLOOD

Leukemia emerges when certain types of white blood cells, known as leukocytes, become cancerous and multiply uncontrollably. These abnormal cells are produced in the bone marrow, the spongy tissue inside our bones responsible for generating new blood cells. As they multiply, the cancerous white blood cells accumulate, crowding out healthy cells and impairing their normal functions. Ultimately, this disrupts the delicate balance within our blood.

THE DOMINO EFFECT

Leukemia possesses the ability to infiltrate and disrupt the normal production of blood cells. As cancerous cells continue to proliferate, they eventually spill into the bloodstream, where they can travel to different parts of the body. This widespread presence of cancer cells can lead to a range of complications, including anemia, bleeding disorders, and increased susceptibility to infections.

IDENTIFYING THE WARNING SIGNS

Detecting leukemia in its early stages can significantly impact treatment outcomes. While symptoms may vary depending on the type and stage of leukemia, common warning signs include:

1. *Fatigue and Weakness.* Persistent feelings of exhaustion, weakness, or a general lack of energy.
2. *Frequent Infections.* Recurrent or severe infections, as the cancerous cells can suppress the normal immune response.
3. *Easy Bruising and Bleeding.* Unexplained bruising, prolonged bleeding from minor cuts, or nosebleeds.
4. *Bone and Joint Pain.* Persistent pain in the bones and joints, often accompanied by tenderness or swelling.
5. *Unexplained Weight Loss.* Sudden and unintentional weight loss, accompanied by a loss of appetite.

DIAGNOSIS AND TREATMENT

Diagnosing leukemia involves a series of tests to determine the type, subtype, and extent of the disease. These tests may include blood tests, bone marrow biopsy, genetic analysis, and imaging studies. Once a diagnosis is confirmed, the healthcare team can develop an individualized treatment plan.

The treatment of leukemia varies depending on several factors, including the type of leukemia, its stage, and the patient's overall health.

BRAIN CANCER: ATTACK ON THE POWERHOUSE

Our brain, the control center of our body, consists of billions of cells called neurons that communicate with each other through electrical signals. These cells work harmoniously, allowing us to think, move, and feel. However, when the normal process of cell growth and division in the brain becomes disrupted, cancerous cells can form, giving rise to brain cancer.

TYPES OF BRAIN CANCER

Brain cancer encompasses a variety of tumor types that can occur within the brain. The two main categories of brain tumors are primary and metastatic.

Primary Brain Tumors. These tumors originate within the brain itself and can be further classified into different types, including gliomas, meningiomas, pituitary tumors, and medulloblastomas. Gliomas, such as astrocytomas and glioblastomas, are the most common primary brain tumors.

Metastatic Brain Tumors. Metastatic brain tumors, also known as secondary brain tumors, occur when cancer cells from other parts of the body, such as the lungs, breasts, or skin, spread to the brain. These tumors are named after the organ from which they originated, rather than the brain itself.

THE OPERATION OF BRAIN CANCER

Brain cancer operates within the intricate network of cells that make up our brain, disrupting its normal functioning. When cancer cells develop in the brain, they grow and multiply, forming a mass called a tumor. As the tumor enlarges, it can exert pressure on the surrounding brain tissue, leading to a range of symptoms and complications.

THE IMPACT OF BRAIN TUMORS

The effects of brain tumors can vary depending on their location, size, and type. Common symptoms associated with brain tumors include:

1. *Headaches.* Persistent or worsening headaches, often accompanied by nausea and vomiting, may be a sign of a brain tumor.
2. *Seizures.* Unexplained seizures or convulsions, which may involve twitching, loss of consciousness, or abnormal sensations.
3. *Cognitive and Behavioral Changes.* Personality changes, memory problems, difficulty concentrating, and mood swings may occur due to brain tumor involvement.
4. *Motor and Sensory Dysfunction.* Weakness or numbness in specific body parts, difficulties with balance or coordination, and changes in vision or hearing.
5. *Speech and Language Problems.* Difficulty speaking or finding the right words, slurred speech, or impaired comprehension.

DIAGNOSIS AND TREATMENT

Diagnosing brain cancer requires a comprehensive evaluation, including imaging tests such as magnetic resonance imaging (MRI) or computed tomography (CT) scans. Additionally, a biopsy may be performed, where a sample of the tumor is extracted and examined under a microscope.

Treatment for brain cancer depends on several factors, including the type, size, and location of the tumor, as well as the overall health of the patient.

PANCREATIC CANCER

The pancreas, a vital organ tucked deep within the abdomen, plays a crucial role in digestion and blood sugar regulation. It produces enzymes that aid in breaking down food and hormones, including insulin, that regulate blood sugar levels. When cancer develops within the pancreas, its normal functions become disrupted.

Pancreatic cancer arises when cells in the pancreas undergo uncontrolled growth, forming a mass or tumor. The majority of pancreatic cancers are adenocarcinomas, originating in the cells that line the pancreatic ducts. These tumors can impede the pancreas' ability to function correctly and may spread to nearby organs and tissues.

Pancreatic cancer often operates silently, remaining undetected until it reaches advanced stages. This is due to the pancreas' location deep within the body, making it difficult to detect early signs or perform routine screenings. Unfortunately, by the time symptoms manifest, the cancer has usually progressed, making treatment more challenging.

IDENTIFYING THE WARNING SIGNS

While pancreatic cancer may not present noticeable symptoms in its early stages, it is important to be vigilant. The following warning signs may indicate a need for further evaluation:

1. *Abdominal Pain.* Persistent or worsening pain in the upper abdomen or back can be a symptom of pancreatic cancer. This pain may radiate and become more severe over time.

2. *Jaundice.* Yellowing of the skin and eyes, accompanied by dark urine and pale stools, may suggest a blockage in the bile ducts caused by pancreatic cancer.

3. *Unexplained Weight Loss.* Sudden and unintentional weight loss, even without changes in diet or exercise, can be a warning sign of pancreatic cancer.

4. *Loss of Appetite.* A significant decrease in appetite and feelings of early satiety, leading to unintended weight loss, may be indicative of pancreatic cancer.

5. *Digestive Problems.* Digestive difficulties such as nausea, vomiting, indigestion, or changes in bowel movements may occur as pancreatic cancer affects the digestive system.

DIAGNOSIS AND TREATMENT

Diagnosing pancreatic cancer requires a comprehensive evaluation, combining medical history, physical examination, imaging tests, and biopsy. Common diagnostic procedures include:

1. *Imaging Tests.* Techniques such as computed tomography (CT) scans, magnetic resonance imaging (MRI), and ultrasound help visualize the pancreas and detect abnormalities or tumors.

2. *Biopsy.* A tissue sample is obtained through a biopsy, either through a fine needle aspiration or surgical procedure, to confirm the presence of cancer cells and determine the specific type of pancreatic cancer.

Once a diagnosis is confirmed, the treatment plan will depend on various factors, including the stage of the cancer, the patient's overall health, and their treatment goals.

CERVICAL CANCER

The cervix is the lower part of the uterus, connecting it to the vagina. It plays a crucial role in the reproductive process, facilitating the passage of menstrual blood and serving as the gateway for sperm during intercourse. The cervix is lined with specialized cells that can undergo changes, sometimes leading to the development of cancer.

Cervical cancer arises when the cells in the cervix undergo abnormal changes, typically caused by persistent infection with certain types of the human papillomavirus (HPV). HPV is a common sexually transmitted infection, and while most cases resolve spontaneously, some infections persist and can lead to the development of cervical cancer over time.

THE DOMINO EFFECT

Cervical cancer operates stealthily, gradually affecting the cells of the cervix and potentially spreading to nearby tissues. If left undetected or untreated, cancer cells can invade the surrounding structures, including the uterus, pelvic wall, and nearby lymph nodes. In advanced stages, cervical cancer may even spread to distant organs, such as the lungs, liver, or bones, impacting overall health.

IDENTIFYING THE WARNING SIGNS

Detecting cervical cancer in its early stages is crucial for successful treatment outcomes. While early cervical cancer may not present noticeable symptoms, the following warning signs may indicate a need for further evaluation:

1. *Abnormal Vaginal Bleeding.* Unusual vaginal bleeding between periods, after intercourse, or after menopause could be a sign of cervical cancer.

2. *Unusual Discharge.* Increased vaginal discharge that is watery, bloody, or has a foul odor should be investigated further.

3. *Pelvic Pain* Persistent or recurring pelvic pain, particularly during intercourse or urination, may be a symptom of advanced cervical cancer.

4. *Painful Intercourse.* Discomfort or pain during sexual intercourse, known as dyspareunia, can be an indication of cervical abnormalities.

5. *Unexplained Weight Loss.* Sudden and unintentional weight loss, without changes in diet or exercise, can sometimes be associated with advanced cervical cancer.

DIAGNOSIS AND TREATMENT

Diagnosing cervical cancer involves a series of tests to assess the presence of abnormal cells and determine the extent of the disease. Common diagnostic procedures include:

1. *Pap Smear.* A Pap smear, also known as a Pap test, involves collecting cells from the cervix to check for any

abnormal changes. This screening test aims to detect precancerous or early-stage cervical cancer.

2. *HPV Test.* This test checks for the presence of high-risk HPV strains in cervical cells, which can increase the risk of developing cervical cancer.

3. *Biopsy.* If abnormalities are detected during a Pap smear or HPV test, a biopsy may be performed. A small tissue sample is collected from the cervix for examination under a microscope to confirm the presence of cancerous cells.

Once a diagnosis is confirmed, the treatment plan will depend on various factors, including the stage of the cancer, the patient's age and overall health, and their desire for future pregnancies.

LIVER CANCER

The liver, a remarkable organ nestled in the upper right abdomen, performs essential functions such as detoxification, metabolism, and bile production. It is composed of different types of cells, including hepatocytes, which can be susceptible to the development of cancer.

Liver cancer, also known as hepatocellular carcinoma (HCC), originates in the hepatocytes—the primary functional cells of the liver. It typically develops as a result of underlying liver diseases, such as chronic hepatitis B or C infection, cirrhosis (scarring of the liver), or excessive alcohol consumption. These conditions can trigger genetic mutations in liver cells, leading to the uncontrolled growth of cancerous cells.

Liver cancer operates within the complex choreography of liver cells, disrupting their normal functions and gradually impacting the organ's structure. As cancerous cells multiply, they form a tumor within the liver. If left unchecked, the tumor can invade nearby tissues and potentially spread to distant organs through the bloodstream or lymphatic system.

IDENTIFYING THE WARNING SIGNS

Detecting liver cancer in its early stages is crucial for successful treatment outcomes. While symptoms may not be evident in the initial phases, the following warning signs may indicate a need for further evaluation:

1. *Abdominal Pain and Swelling.* Persistent pain or discomfort in the upper abdomen, accompanied by abdominal swelling or a feeling of fullness, may indicate liver cancer.

2. *Unexplained Weight Loss.* Sudden and unintentional weight loss, even without changes in diet or physical activity, can be a warning sign of liver cancer.

3. *Jaundice.* Yellowing of the skin and eyes, along with dark urine and pale stools, may indicate liver dysfunction caused by liver cancer.

4. *Fatigue and Weakness.* Persistent fatigue, weakness, and a general decline in energy levels may be associated with liver cancer.

5. *Digestive Issues.* Nausea, vomiting, loss of appetite, and changes in bowel habits can occur as liver cancer affects the digestive system.

Please remember that if you experience any of these symptoms or have concerns about your liver health, it is crucial to consult a healthcare professional for further evaluation and appropriate testing.

DIAGNOSIS AND TREATMENT

Diagnosing liver cancer requires a comprehensive evaluation, including medical history, physical examination, imaging tests, and blood tests. Common diagnostic procedures include:

1. *Imaging Tests.* Techniques such as ultrasound, computed tomography (CT) scans, and magnetic resonance imaging (MRI) help visualize the liver and detect any abnormalities or tumors.
2. *Blood Tests.* Blood tests can measure levels of certain proteins and enzymes that indicate liver function and detect tumor markers associated with liver cancer.
3. *Biopsy.* A tissue sample is obtained through a biopsy, either with a needle or during surgery, to confirm the presence of cancer cells and determine the specific type of liver cancer.

Once a diagnosis is confirmed, the treatment plan will depend on various factors, including the stage of the cancer, the patient's overall health, and their treatment goals.

OTHER TYPES OF CANCER

While we have explored some of the most common types of cancer, it is important to acknowledge that cancer can manifest in various other parts of the body. These include ovarian cancer, kidney cancer and bladder cancer, among others. Each type has its own unique characteristics, risk factors, and treatment approaches.

STAGES OF CANCER: NAVIGATING THE LANDSCAPE

Within the realm of cancer, staging is the cartographer's art—an intricate process that maps the terrain of the disease, guiding patients and their healthcare team on the path to recovery. From stage I, where cancer is confined to its birthplace, to the more advanced stages where it ventures beyond its original borders, staging provides a compass, guiding treatment decisions and prognostic expectations. Fear not the stage, for knowledge empowers, and hope springs eternal.

The staging of cancer involves determining the size and extent of the primary tumor, the involvement of nearby lymph nodes, and the presence or absence of distant metastasis. This information is crucial for devising an individualized treatment plan and estimating the prognosis. Staging systems differ for various types of cancer, but they share the common goal of providing a standardized framework for assessing the extent of disease.

THE SIGNIFICANCE OF CANCER STAGING

Before we embark on our journey, it is important to understand the significance of cancer staging. Imagine standing at the starting point of an unfamiliar path, unsure of the terrain ahead. Cancer staging is like a map, providing crucial information about the disease's progression, potential spread, and treatment options. By determining the stage of cancer, we gain valuable insights into prognosis, guiding both patients and healthcare professionals in making informed decisions regarding treatment and care.

STAGE 0: THE INCEPTION OF ABNORMALITY

Our journey begins with stage 0—a stage that signifies the inception of abnormal cell growth. At this stage, the cancer is confined to the site of origin, without spreading to nearby tissues or organs. Stage 0 cancers are often referred to as carcinoma in situ, meaning "cancer in place." The abnormal cells are present but have not invaded the surrounding healthy tissues. Early detection and treatment at this stage offer an excellent chance of complete recovery.

STAGE I: THE EMERGING BATTLEFRONT

As we progress to stage I, the battle against cancer intensifies. At this point, the tumor has started to grow and invade nearby tissues, but its reach remains limited. The cancer is still localized, with no evidence of spread to lymph nodes or distant organs. Stage I cancers are typically smaller in size and have a favorable prognosis. Treatment options may include surgery to remove the tumor, radiation therapy, and, in some cases, targeted therapy or chemotherapy.

STAGE II: EXPANDING HORIZONS

In stage II, the battlefront expands, and the cancer grows further, infiltrating adjacent tissues. While the cancer is still localized, it may have a higher risk of spreading to nearby lymph nodes. Stage II cancers require comprehensive treatment approaches, which often include surgery, radiation therapy, and sometimes chemotherapy or targeted therapy. The goal is to eliminate the cancerous cells and reduce the risk of further spread.

STAGE III: THE INFILTRATION SPREADS

As we advance to stage III, cancer reveals its infiltrative nature. It has breached the boundaries of the primary site and invaded nearby lymph nodes. The potential for metastasis, or the spread to distant organs, becomes more significant. Stage III cancers often require a multidisciplinary treatment approach, including surgery, radiation therapy, chemotherapy, targeted therapy, and sometimes immunotherapy. The aim is to eliminate cancer cells both at the primary site and in the affected lymph nodes.

STAGE IV: THE JOURNEY OF METASTASIS

In stage IV, we confront the journey of metastasis—the point at which cancer cells break away from the primary tumor, traveling through the bloodstream or lymphatic system to establish colonies in distant organs. Stage IV cancer is considered advanced, and the treatment approach focuses on controlling the disease, managing symptoms, and improving quality of life. Treatment options may include surgery to remove the primary tumor and palliative measures such as radiation therapy, chemotherapy, targeted therapy, and immunotherapy. While stage IV cancers are generally not curable, advancements in treatments have improved outcomes and prolonged survival for many patients.

TNM SYSTEM: DECODING THE LANGUAGE OF CANCER STAGING

To effectively communicate the stage of cancer, healthcare professionals use a standardized system called the TNM system. This system utilizes three key factors to categorize the disease:

TUMOR (T)

The T factor describes the size and extent of the primary tumor, ranging from T0 (no evidence of a tumor) to T4 (a large tumor that has invaded nearby structures).

NODE (N)

The N factor indicates the involvement of nearby lymph nodes, ranging from N0 (no involvement) to N3 (extensive lymph node involvement). The presence or absence of cancer in the lymph nodes provides crucial information about the potential spread of the disease.

METASTASIS (M)

The M factor signifies whether the cancer has spread to distant organs. It ranges from M0 (no evidence of metastasis) to M1 (presence of distant metastasis). Understanding the extent of metastasis is crucial in determining the stage of cancer.

By combining these elements, healthcare professionals assign a stage to the cancer, ranging from 0 to IV, facilitating clear communication and guiding treatment decisions.

As we continue our voyage, we will dive deeper into the treatment options available for each stage, exploring the advancements in surgery, radiation therapy, chemotherapy, targeted therapy, immunotherapy, and supportive care. Remember, no matter the stage, there is always hope. Together, we will navigate the challenges, conquer the obstacles, and forge ahead on the path toward recovery and healing.

TREATMENT OPTIONS: A MULTIFACETED SYMPHONY

In the battle against cancer, a symphony of treatment options plays out—a harmonious collaboration of medical expertise, cutting-edge research, and unwavering determination. Surgery, radiation therapy, chemotherapy, immunotherapy— each note in this melodious ensemble has its role to play. With every treatment option, hope is kindled, and the potential for a triumphant crescendo draws closer.

Before we dive into the specifics of treatment options, it is crucial to understand the overarching goals of cancer treatment. The primary objectives include:

Curative Treatment. The eradication of cancer cells with the intent of achieving a complete cure.

Palliative Treatment. The management of symptoms and improvement of the patient's quality of life, particularly in cases where a cure is not feasible.

Adjuvant Treatment. Additional therapy given after the primary treatment, such as surgery, to reduce the risk of cancer recurrence.

Neoadjuvant Treatment. Treatment administered before the primary therapy, often done to shrink tumors, making surgery or other treatments more effective.

The treatment landscape for cancer is vast and multifaceted, with each modality targeting different aspects of the disease. Let us explore the most common treatment options and their roles in the fight against cancer

SURGERY

Surgery is a time-tested and essential treatment modality in the fight against cancer. It involves the physical removal of cancerous tissue from the body, aiming to eliminate the tumor and any nearby affected tissue. Let's explore how surgery takes effect on a cellular level and the advantages it offers.

MECHANISM OF ACTION

During surgery, the surgeon carefully removes the tumor along with a margin of surrounding healthy tissue. This margin is crucial to ensure complete removal of cancer cells. Depending on the location and size of the tumor, different surgical approaches may be employed, including open surgery, minimally invasive procedures, or robot-assisted surgery. The goal is to remove all visible cancer cells, reducing the risk of recurrence.

ADVANTAGES OF SURGERY

Curative Intent: Surgery can be curative for localized cancers, where the disease has not spread beyond its site of origin. It offers the potential for complete removal of the tumor, leading to a cure.

1. *Immediate Results.* Surgery provides immediate results by physically removing the tumor, providing relief and peace of mind for patients and their loved ones.
2. *Staging and Diagnosis.* Surgical procedures can help determine the stage and extent of cancer, aiding in treatment planning and decision-making.

3. *Symptom Relief.* In some cases, surgery can alleviate symptoms caused by the tumor, such as pain, obstruction, or bleeding.

POTENTIAL SIDE EFFECTS

1. *Pain and Discomfort.* After surgery, patients may experience pain and discomfort at the incision site, which can be managed with appropriate pain medications.
2. *Infection.* There is a risk of developing an infection at the surgical site. It is important to follow post-operative care instructions and report any signs of infection, such as redness, swelling, or drainage.
3. *Scarring.* Surgery leaves a scar at the incision site, which varies in size and appearance depending on the surgical approach and individual healing process.
4. *Functional Changes.* Depending on the location and extent of surgery, there may be functional changes or limitations. For example, removal of certain organs or tissues may impact bodily functions or require rehabilitation.

RADIATION THERAPY

Radiation therapy utilizes high-energy beams, such as X-rays or protons, to destroy cancer cells and shrink tumors. It can be delivered externally (external beam radiation) or internally (brachytherapy).

MECHANISM OF ACTION

Radiation therapy damages the DNA of cancer cells, impairing their ability to divide and grow. This damage is done with precision, targeting the tumor while minimizing exposure to nearby healthy tissues. The goal is to kill cancer cells and shrink tumors, either as a primary treatment or in combination with other modalities.

ADVANTAGES OF RADIATION THERAPY

1. *Localized Treatment.* Radiation therapy is localized to the treatment area, allowing precise targeting of cancer cells while minimizing damage to healthy tissues.

2. *Preserving Organ Function.* In some cases, radiation therapy can help preserve organ function by reducing tumor size or preventing tumor growth.

3. *Adjuvant Therapy.* Radiation therapy can be used as adjuvant therapy after surgery to kill any remaining cancer cells in the area and reduce the risk of recurrence.

4. *Palliative Care.* Radiation therapy can be used to alleviate symptoms, such as pain or obstruction, by shrinking tumors or reducing their impact on surrounding tissues.

POTENTIAL SIDE EFFECTS

1. *Fatigue.* Radiation therapy can cause fatigue, which can accumulate over the course of treatment. Resting and conserving energy is important during this time.

2. *Skin Changes.* Radiation therapy can cause skin reactions in the treatment area, ranging from redness and dryness to blistering and peeling. Proper skincare and following the healthcare team's recommendations are essential.

3. *Temporary Hair Loss.* Depending on the location of radiation therapy, temporary hair loss may occur in the treatment area. Hair usually regrows after treatment.

4. *Long-term Effects.* In some cases, radiation therapy may have long-term effects on surrounding tissues or organs, such as fibrosis or secondary cancers. These risks are carefully weighed against the potential benefits.

CHEMOTHERAPY

Chemotherapy, often referred to as "chemo," is a systemic treatment that involves the use of drugs to kill cancer cells or inhibit their growth. It works by targeting rapidly dividing cells, which includes both cancer cells and some healthy cells.

MECHANISM OF ACTION

Chemotherapy drugs are designed to interfere with the ability of cancer cells to divide and grow. They can be administered orally or intravenously and travel throughout the body via the bloodstream. These drugs target cancer cells wherever they may be, attacking them at different stages of the cell cycle.

ADVANTAGES OF CHEMOTHERAPY

1. *Systemic Treatment.* Chemotherapy can reach cancer cells throughout the body, making it a valuable option for cancers that have spread or cannot be easily treated with surgery or radiation therapy alone.

2. *Adjuvant Therapy.* Chemotherapy can be used as adjuvant therapy after surgery to kill any remaining cancer cells and reduce the risk of recurrence.

3. *Combination Therapy.* Chemotherapy can be combined with other treatment modalities, such as surgery or radiation therapy, to improve treatment outcomes.

4. *Palliative Care.* In cases where a cure is not possible, chemotherapy can be used to shrink tumors, alleviate symptoms, and improve the patient's quality of life.

POTENTIAL SIDE EFFECTS

1. *Hair Loss.* Chemotherapy affects rapidly dividing cells, including hair follicles, leading to hair loss. This can be temporary, and hair usually grows back after treatment.

2. *Nausea and Vomiting.* Some chemotherapy drugs can cause nausea and vomiting. Medications called antiemetics can help manage these side effects.

3. *Fatigue.* Chemotherapy can cause fatigue, which can range from mild to severe. It is important to balance rest and activity and seek support from healthcare professionals.

4. *Weakened Immune System.* Chemotherapy can suppress the immune system, making individuals more susceptible to infections. Taking precautions and practicing good hygiene is essential.

TARGETED THERAPY

Targeted therapy represents a revolution in cancer treatment, aiming to disrupt specific molecular targets that drive cancer growth and survival. Let's explore how targeted therapy takes effect on a cellular level and the advantages it offers:

MECHANISM OF ACTION

Targeted therapy drugs are designed to identify and block specific molecules or pathways that are crucial for cancer cell growth and survival. By inhibiting these targets, targeted therapy can impede cancer progression and shrink tumors. Different targeted therapies may work by interfering with the signaling pathways, inhibiting angiogenesis (formation of new blood vessels to support tumor growth), or directly attacking specific mutated proteins within cancer cells.

ADVANTAGES OF TARGETED THERAPY

1. *Precision Treatment.* Targeted therapy is designed to specifically target cancer cells, minimizing harm to healthy cells and reducing side effects compared to traditional chemotherapy.

2. *Personalized Medicine.* Targeted therapy is tailored to the individual's specific cancer type and genetic profile. Molecular testing helps identify the molecular targets and guide treatment decisions.

3. *Increased Treatment Efficacy.* Targeted therapy has demonstrated remarkable effectiveness in certain cancer types, leading to tumor shrinkage, improved outcomes, and prolonged survival.

4. *Combination Potential.* Targeted therapy can be used alone or in combination with other treatment modalities, such as chemotherapy or radiation therapy, to enhance treatment outcomes.

IMMUNOTHERAPY

Immunotherapy represents a groundbreaking approach that harnesses the power of the immune system to recognize and attack cancer cells.

MECHANISM OF ACTION

Immunotherapy aims to enhance the body's natural defense mechanisms against cancer. It involves the use of substances, such as immune checkpoint inhibitors or CAR-T cell therapy, which stimulate or enhance the immune response against cancer cells. These therapies can either unleash the brakes on the immune system or genetically modify immune cells to specifically target cancer cells.

ADVANTAGES OF IMMUNOTHERAPY

1. *Enhanced Immune Response.* Immunotherapy helps activate or boost the immune system, enabling it to recognize and attack cancer cells more effectively.

2. *Long-Term Response.* Some immunotherapy treatments have shown durable responses, with the potential for long-term remission or even cure in certain cases.

3. *Broader Applicability.* Immunotherapy has demonstrated effectiveness across a range of cancer types, including melanoma, lung cancer, kidney cancer, and more.

4. *Combination Potential.* Immunotherapy can be used in combination with other treatments, such as chemotherapy or targeted therapy, to enhance treatment effectiveness.

POTENTIAL SIDE EFFECTS

Immune-related Adverse Events: Immunotherapy can lead to immune-related side effects, known as immune-related adverse events. These may include fatigue, skin rashes, diarrhea, or inflammation of organs such as the lungs, liver, or thyroid. Prompt recognition and management of these side effects are crucial.

PRECISION MEDICINE

Precision medicine represents a paradigm shift in cancer treatment, focusing on individualized care based on a person's genetic profile and specific tumor characteristics.

MECHANISM OF ACTION

Precision medicine utilizes molecular testing, such as genetic sequencing, to identify specific genetic mutations or alterations within cancer cells. This information is used to guide treatment decisions, selecting therapies that target these specific mutations or pathways. Precision medicine may involve targeted therapies, immunotherapies, or other innovative treatments.

ADVANTAGES OF PRECISION MEDICINE

1. *Personalized Treatment.* Precision medicine allows for tailored treatment plans based on the unique genetic makeup of an individual's cancer cells.

2. *Improved Treatment Efficacy.* By targeting specific genetic alterations driving cancer growth, precision medicine can increase treatment effectiveness and potentially enhance outcomes.

3. *Reduced Side Effects.* Precision medicine's targeted approach aims to minimize harm to healthy cells, thereby reducing side effects compared to conventional treatments.

4. *Clinical Trial Opportunities.* Precision medicine opens doors to participation in clinical trials exploring novel targeted therapies or immunotherapies, providing access to cutting-edge treatments.

POTENTIAL SIDE EFFECTS

Similar to targeted therapy and immunotherapy, the potential side effects of precision medicine depend on the specific treatment modality employed. Monitoring and management of treatment-related side effects remain important components of patient care.

TREATMENT CONSIDERATIONS FOR DIFFERENT STAGES OF CANCER

The choice of treatment options may vary depending on the stage of cancer.

EARLY-STAGE CANCER

In the early stages of cancer, when the disease is localized and has not spread beyond its site of origin, the primary goal is often curative treatment. Surgery is typically the mainstay treatment, aiming to remove the tumor and any nearby affected tissue. In some cases, adjuvant therapy, such as radiation therapy or chemotherapy, may be recommended to reduce the risk of recurrence.

ADVANCED OR METASTATIC CANCER

When cancer has spread to other parts of the body, the focus shifts to palliative treatment, which aims to alleviate symptoms, improve quality of life, and extend survival. Treatment options may include surgery, radiation therapy, chemotherapy, targeted therapy, immunotherapy, or a combination thereof. The choice of treatment depends on several factors, including the specific cancer type, the extent of metastasis, the individual's overall health, and their treatment preferences.

RECURRENT CANCER

In cases of cancer recurrence, where the disease returns after a period of remission, treatment options depend on several factors, including the location and extent of recurrence, previous treatments received, and the individual's overall health. Treatment options may involve surgery, radiation therapy, chemotherapy, targeted therapy, immunotherapy, or participation in clinical trials.

THE DIAGNOSIS

The moment of receiving a cancer diagnosis can be a profound and life-altering experience. It is a moment that forever marks the beginning of a transformative journey, filled with uncertainties, challenges, and, most importantly, hope.

The journey of a cancer diagnosis often begins with the recognition of signs and symptoms that raise concerns. As earlier discussed, these can vary depending on the type of cancer. It is crucial to pay attention to these signs and seek medical attention if they persist or worsen.

Upon recognizing concerning signs or symptoms, the next step is to seek a medical consultation. This typically involves scheduling an appointment with a primary care physician or a specialist, such as an oncologist. The healthcare provider will conduct a comprehensive evaluation, which may include a detailed medical history, physical examination, and order additional diagnostic tests.

Imaging studies play a vital role in cancer diagnosis, providing detailed visualizations of the internal structures of the body. Laboratory tests are also essential in diagnosing cancer, as they provide insights into the composition of bodily fluids and tissues. Blood tests, such as complete blood counts, tumor markers, and genetic tests, can help detect abnormalities, assess organ function, and identify specific genetic mutations or alterations associated with certain cancers.

A biopsy is often the definitive step in cancer diagnosis. It involves the removal of a small tissue sample from a suspicious area, which is then examined under a microscope by a pathologist. The analysis of the biopsy sample helps determine the presence of cancer, its type, grade, and stage, guiding subsequent treatment decisions.

Staging, the detailed analysis to provide critical information about the extent of the disease, and grading, the assessment of the cellular characteristics of cancer cells, helps determine the aggressiveness and potential for spreading of the cancer.

The diagnosis of cancer marks the beginning of a profound and transformative journey. By understanding the diagnostic process, seeking timely medical attention, and embracing emotional support, individuals can navigate this path with courage, resilience, and hope.

PART I

Laying the Foundation for Healing

2

THE SHOCK OF A CANCER DIAGNOSIS

A cancer diagnosis is a seismic event that can shake a person's world to its core. The news can send shockwaves through every aspect of their being, leaving them reeling from the sudden disruption of their life's trajectory.

When a person first receives a cancer diagnosis, the initial impact can be overwhelming. They may experience a range of emotions, from disbelief and denial to fear and sadness. The mind struggles to process the reality of the situation, grappling with the idea that their own body has become a battlefield where cancer cells threaten their well-being. Denial serves as a protective mechanism, allowing individuals time to absorb the shock at their own pace.

Fear and anxiety become constant companions in the wake of a cancer diagnosis. Thoughts of mortality and uncertainty about the future may haunt their every waking moment. The fear of the unknown takes hold, overshadowing the once-familiar landscape of their life. It is important to recognize that fear is a natural response, and it is crucial to address these fears with compassion and support.

The diagnosis of cancer often brings about a deep sense of sadness and grief. Individuals mourn the loss of their pre-diagnosis life, the dreams and plans they had envisioned, and the sense of control they once had over their own body. It is vital to acknowledge these emotions and allow oneself to grieve. Finding solace in the support of loved ones or seeking professional counseling can provide a safe space to process these emotions and work towards acceptance.

Coping with the shock of a cancer diagnosis involves engaging in cognitive processing. The mind tirelessly tries to make sense of the situation, seeking answers, and grasping for a sense of understanding. Thoughts related to the diagnosis, treatment options, and potential outcomes may consume the mind. Intrusive thoughts and a constant need for information become a part of everyday life. It is essential to give oneself time and space to process these thoughts, seeking support when needed, and finding a balance between seeking knowledge and allowing oneself moments of respite.

Emotional processing is another crucial aspect of navigating the shock of a cancer diagnosis. It involves acknowledging and expressing the multitude of emotions that arise. Fear, anger, sadness, and vulnerability may coexist within an individual's emotional landscape. It is important to create a safe and supportive environment to explore and process these emotions. Journaling, talking to trusted loved ones, or seeking the guidance of a professional counselor can provide avenues for emotional release and healing.

A cancer diagnosis often brings about a reevaluation of one's identity and self-concept. Questions of self-worth, body image, and the role one plays in relationships and society may arise. The sudden shift in circumstances challenges the individual's sense of self and may leave them feeling vulnerable and unsure. It is essential to nurture self-compassion and to remember that one's worth is not defined by the presence of cancer.

Finding ways to embrace the journey of a cancer diagnosis is a deeply personal and individual process. Acceptance becomes a cornerstone of this journey. It involves acknowledging the reality of the diagnosis and finding ways to face it head-on. Acceptance does not imply resignation or giving up, but rather the recognition of the need to confront the situation with courage and resilience. Adopting a positive mindset, cultivating gratitude, and nurturing optimism then comes into play in shifting one's perspective and paving the way for healing and growth.

Seeking support from loved ones, healthcare professionals, support groups, or therapists is instrumental in navigating the shock of a cancer diagnosis. Surrounding oneself with a network of understanding and compassionate individuals can provide strength and guidance. Sharing experiences, fears, and triumphs with others who have walked a similar path can also foster connection and a sense of belonging. Seeking support allows individuals to feel heard, validated, and empowered in their journey.

Self-care becomes paramount in the face of a cancer diagnosis. It involves tending to one's physical, emotional, and spiritual well-being. Here, prioritizing rest, relaxation, and engaging in activities that bring joy and fulfillment are crucial for maintaining a sense of balance. Self-care empowers individuals to take an active role in their healing journey and regain a sense of control amidst the uncertainties.

Redefining priorities and finding meaning are transformative aspects of embracing the journey of a cancer diagnosis. The diagnosis serves as a catalyst for reflecting on what truly matters in life. It is an opportunity to forge deeper connections with loved ones, seek out new passions, and pursue a life filled with purpose and meaning. Finding meaning amidst this adversity allows individuals to channel their energy into personal growth and transcend the limitations imposed by cancer.

3

THE MIND-BODY CONNECTION

In the realm of healing, an extraordinary connection exists between the mind and the body. It is a connection that transcends the boundaries of conventional medicine, harnessing the power of our thoughts, emotions, and beliefs to shape our physical well-being. This connection, known as the mind-body connection, holds immense potential for those facing the challenges of cancer.

Imagine for a moment a world where our thoughts possess the power to shape our reality, where our inner landscape, rich with hope, resilience, and positivity, serves as a potent force in healing. This is the realm we venture into— a realm that holds the promise of enhancing our well-being and empowering us to navigate the challenging path of cancer with grace and strength.

Throughout history, the interplay between the mind and the body has been recognized and explored by ancient healing traditions, spiritual practices, and pioneering minds. Today, scientific research continues to unravel the intricate mechanisms through which our mental and emotional states can influence our physical health and healing processes.

Understanding the mind-body connection is not about disregarding the essential role of medical interventions in cancer treatment. Instead, it is about recognizing that the mind is a powerful ally, capable of influencing our experiences and outcomes. It is about embracing a holistic approach to healing that integrates the best of both worlds—medical science and the power of the mind.

The mind-body connection is not a mystical concept reserved for a select few. It is a profound truth that resides within each and every one of us. It is the recognition and cultivation of this innate power that can ignite the spark of transformation within us.

The mind's influence on the healing process is a symphony of interconnected factors. Our thoughts, beliefs, and attitudes orchestrate a symphony of biochemical and physiological responses within our bodies. Scientific research has shed light on the intricate ways in which the mind can modulate the immune system, reduce stress, and optimize the body's natural healing mechanisms.

In the bustling chaos of modern life, cultivating mindful awareness becomes a transformative practice in navigating the challenges of cancer. By anchoring our attention in the present moment, we can foster a deep connection with our bodies, nurturing self-compassion and resilience. Mindfulness allows us to observe our thoughts and emotions without judgment, unlocking the potential to respond to cancer with grace, strength, and clarity.

While the healing power of the mind does not claim to be a standalone cure, it can be an invaluable ally in the journey through cancer. By harnessing the mind's potential, we can cultivate a supportive environment that complements conventional medical treatments, empowering us to actively participate in our healing process. As you embark on this journey, remember that the mind and body are partners, capable of orchestrating a symphony of healing. Embrace the power of the mind-body connection, and discover the transformative potential that resides within you.

NEUROPLASTICITY AND HEALING: REWIRING THE BRAIN FOR RECOVERY

The human brain is a marvelous organ that possesses an extraordinary ability to adapt and change throughout our lives. This capacity, known as neuroplasticity, has captivated scientists and medical professionals for decades. In recent years, the concept of neuroplasticity has gained significant attention in the field of medicine, particularly in understanding how it can contribute to healing and recovery from various health conditions, including cancer.

Neuroplasticity refers to the brain's remarkable ability to reorganize itself, forming new neural connections and modifying existing ones. This process occurs in response to our experiences, thoughts, emotions, and even physical changes. It allows the brain to adapt, learn, and recover from injuries or diseases.

At its core, neuroplasticity is driven by the brain's fundamental building blocks: neurons. Neurons are the specialized cells responsible for transmitting information in the form of electrical impulses. They communicate through intricate networks of synapses, which are the connections between neurons. These synapses allow information to flow and create the foundation for our thoughts, emotions, and behaviors.

Neuroplasticity operates through various mechanisms, each contributing to the brain's ability to rewire itself. One key mechanism is synaptic plasticity, which involves strengthening or weakening the connections between neurons. When we repeatedly engage in a specific activity or thought pattern, the synapses associated with that activity become stronger, facilitating more efficient communication between neurons.

Another mechanism is structural plasticity, which refers to the brain's capacity to physically change its structure. It involves the growth of new neurons, the formation of new connections between neurons, and even the rewiring of existing pathways. Through structural plasticity, the brain can adapt and compensate for injuries or changes in its environment.

THE ROLE OF NEUROPLASTICITY IN HEALING

Now, let us delve into the captivating role of neuroplasticity in the healing process, particularly in the context of cancer. When individuals are diagnosed with cancer, it can be a physically and emotionally challenging experience. Cancer treatments, such as surgery, chemotherapy, and radiation therapy, can also impact the brain and its functioning. This is where the power of neuroplasticity comes into play.

In the face of cancer and its treatments, the brain has the potential to undergo transformative changes that support healing and recovery. Neuroplasticity allows the brain to adapt to the new circumstances, compensate for any damage, and optimize its functioning. For example, if a particular brain area is affected by surgery or radiation therapy, other regions can step in and assume the lost functions, a phenomenon known as functional reorganization.

Furthermore, neuroplasticity enables the brain to mitigate the cognitive changes often associated with cancer and its treatments, such as memory loss, attention difficulties, and executive function impairments. Through the formation of new neural connections and the strengthening of existing ones, individuals can experience improvements in cognitive abilities, memory retrieval, and overall cognitive functioning.

HARNESSING NEUROPLASTICITY FOR RECOVERY

The question arises: How can we harness the power of neuroplasticity to support healing and recovery? The answer lies in engaging in activities and practices that stimulate and optimize neuroplasticity.

1. *Cognitive Stimulation.* Engaging in mentally stimulating activities, such as puzzles, reading, and learning new skills, can promote neuroplasticity. These activities challenge the brain and encourage the formation of new connections, enhancing cognitive function and supporting recovery.

2. *Physical Exercise.* Physical exercise has been shown to have a profound impact on neuroplasticity. Aerobic exercises, strength training, and activities that challenge balance and coordination promote the growth of new neurons and the formation of neural connections. Regular exercise not only supports brain health but also improves mood and overall well-being.

3. *Mindfulness and Meditation.* Practices like mindfulness and meditation have been found to enhance neuroplasticity. By cultivating present-moment awareness and reducing stress, these practices can positively influence the brain's ability to adapt and recover. Mindfulness-based interventions have shown promising results in mitigating treatment-related symptoms and improving overall quality of life.

4. *Rehabilitation Therapies.* Rehabilitation therapies, such as physical therapy, occupational therapy, and speech therapy, can also leverage neuroplasticity for recovery. These therapies aim to retrain and strengthen specific neural pathways, facilitating the restoration of lost functions and promoting independence.

5. *Optimizing Sleep.* Sleep is essential for brain health and neuroplasticity. Quality sleep supports the consolidation of memories, facilitates the removal of toxins, and promotes overall brain recovery. Establishing healthy sleep habits and creating a conducive sleep environment can optimize the brain's healing capacity.

6. *Cultivating a Healing Mindset.* The mind has a profound influence on neuroplasticity. Cultivating a positive mindset, embracing hope, and nurturing resilience can enhance the brain's ability to adapt and recover. Practices such as positive affirmations, visualization, and self-compassion contribute to a healing mindset and support neuroplasticity.

Neuroplasticity is a fascinating concept that holds great promise for healing and recovery. Understanding the brain's capacity to rewire itself opens up exciting possibilities for individuals facing the challenges of cancer and other health conditions. By actively engaging in activities that stimulate neuroplasticity, individuals can support their own healing journey and optimize their chances of regaining lost functions, improving cognitive abilities, and enhancing overall well-being. Neuroplasticity reminds us that our brains possess incredible potential, and with the right approach, we can harness this power to promote healing, resilience, and a better quality of life.

4

OVERCOMING FEAR AND DOUBT: EMBRACING HOPE AND RESILIENCE

Fear is an innate human response to perceived danger or threat. When it comes to cancer, fear can manifest in various ways, such as anxiety, worry, and a sense of uncertainty. It is essential to recognize and understand fear to address its impact on our overall well-being.

Fear can have a profound impact on our mental, emotional, and physical health. It can lead to increased stress levels, which, in turn, can weaken our immune system and hinder the body's ability to heal. By understanding fear and its potential consequences, we can take proactive steps to manage and alleviate it.

The first step in understanding fear is acknowledging its presence in our lives. By acknowledging our fears, we can begin to examine them more closely and understand their underlying causes. Is it the fear of the unknown, the fear of pain, or the fear of losing control? Identifying the specific fears that arise from a cancer diagnosis can help us address them more effectively.

Another key element in overcoming fear and doubt is shifting our perspectives. It involves reframing our thoughts and beliefs surrounding cancer, moving from a place of fear to a place of empowerment. By viewing cancer as an opportunity for growth, resilience, and self-discovery, we open ourselves up to new possibilities and strengths that lie within us.

Seeking support also plays an important role in overcoming the fear associated with a cancer diagnosis. Navigating the complexities of cancer can be daunting, and it is crucial to seek support from loved ones, healthcare professionals, and support groups. By sharing our fears and doubts with trusted individuals, we can gain a fresh perspective, validation, and encouragement. Connecting with others who have walked a similar path can provide invaluable support, guidance, and reassurance. Always remember, you do not have to face cancer alone.

Expressing our fears, doubts, and emotions through creative outlets such as writing, art, or music can be incredibly liberating. It provides an avenue for self-expression and can serve as a cathartic release. Engaging in creative activities allows us to process our emotions, gain clarity, and find solace. Embracing self-expression empowers us to acknowledge and transcend our fears, transforming them into sources of strength and inspiration.

Cancer often brings uncertainty into our lives, and learning to embrace it is a powerful way to overcome fear and doubt. Rather than resisting uncertainty, we can approach it with curiosity and openness. Embracing uncertainty allows us to let go of the need for absolute control and trust in the journey ahead. It is through embracing the unknown that we find the strength to face our fears and doubts with a sense of courage and resilience.

Overcoming fear and doubt is a profound aspect of the mind's power in battling cancer. Remember, you have the power within you to rise above fear and doubt, to embrace your journey with courage, and to find hope and healing along the way. Trust in your ability to overcome, and let your mind be a source of unwavering support and resilience. In the battle of overcoming our fears, cultivating the values of hope and resilience are also of vital importance.

TAMING THE INNER CRITIC: HARNESSING SELF-COMPASSION

Battling cancer is a journey filled with challenges, both physical and emotional. During this time, it is common for our inner critic to become more active, amplifying self-doubt, blame, and harsh self-judgment. However, learning to tame the inner critic and cultivate self-compassion can be a powerful tool in our fight against cancer.

The inner critic is that voice inside our heads that often criticizes and judges us harshly. It can be relentless, feeding us negative thoughts and beliefs about ourselves. When facing a cancer diagnosis, the inner critic can become even more active, heightening feelings of guilt, shame, and self-blame.

It is important to recognize that the inner critic is not our true voice. It is a product of our conditioning, shaped by societal expectations, past experiences, and the pressures we place on ourselves. Understanding this distinction is the first step towards taming the inner critic.

Taming the inner critic involves developing awareness of its presence and consciously challenging its negative messages. It requires cultivating self-compassion and nurturing a kinder and more understanding inner dialogue.

One effective strategy to tame the inner critic is practicing mindfulness. By bringing our attention to the present moment and observing our thoughts without judgment, we can create distance from the inner critic's voice. Mindfulness allows us to recognize that we are not defined by our thoughts and that we have the power to choose how we respond to them.

Another powerful technique is reframing our self-talk. When the inner critic starts to berate us, we can consciously challenge those negative thoughts and replace them with positive and affirming statements. For example, if the inner critic says, "You're not strong enough to beat this," we can counter with, "I am resilient, and I have the strength to face this challenge."

HARNESSING SELF-COMPASSION

Self-compassion is the practice of treating ourselves with kindness, understanding, and acceptance, especially during difficult times. It involves extending the same empathy and compassion we would offer to a loved one to ourselves.

When battling cancer, self-compassion becomes even more critical. It allows us to acknowledge our pain, fear, and vulnerability without judgment. It reminds us that it is normal to struggle and experience a range of emotions during this journey.

To cultivate self-compassion, we can start by practicing self-care. This includes engaging in activities that nurture our physical, emotional, and mental well-being. Taking time to rest, practicing relaxation techniques, engaging in hobbies, and seeking support from loved ones are all important acts of self-compassion.

Additionally, it is essential to practice self-forgiveness. Cancer can bring about a range of emotions, including guilt or regret about past choices or behaviors. However, holding onto these feelings only adds to our burden. By forgiving ourselves for perceived shortcomings or mistakes, we can free ourselves from unnecessary guilt and self-blame.

Embracing self-compassion also means recognizing our strengths and acknowledging our efforts. Celebrating small victories and giving ourselves credit for the steps we take in our cancer journey fosters a sense of self-worth and resilience.

By recognizing the presence of the inner critic, challenging negative self-talk, and embracing self-compassion, we can create a nurturing and supportive inner environment that enhances our well-being and treatment outcomes.

CULTIVATING FAITH IN THE HEALING PROCESS: TRUSTING THE JOURNEY

Faith, in this context, is not limited to religious beliefs, but rather a deep trust in the journey towards healing and the profound influence of the mind-body connection. It encompasses the belief that our bodies possess an innate capacity to heal and restore balance. It recognizes the interconnectedness of our physical, mental, and emotional well-being and acknowledges that our thoughts, beliefs, and emotions can influence our overall health.

Cultivating faith in the healing process does not imply disregarding medical advice or treatments. Instead, it involves integrating a positive mindset and belief in the body's remarkable ability to heal alongside medical interventions. It is about embracing a holistic approach that harmonizes medical expertise with the power of the mind.

TRUSTING THE JOURNEY

Trusting the journey of healing requires a fundamental shift in perspective. It means acknowledging that while we may not have control over the ultimate outcome, we have the power to shape our response and navigate the challenges that accompany cancer treatment.

One crucial aspect of trusting the journey involves developing a strong rapport with your healthcare team. It is essential to have confidence in their expertise, experience, and commitment to your well-being. Establishing open lines of communication and engaging in shared decision-making instills a sense of security and fosters trust in the treatment process.

Trusting the journey also necessitates cultivating confidence in your own intuition and inner wisdom. Each person's cancer journey is unique, and what works for one may not work for another. By trusting yourself and embracing your body's wisdom, you can make informed decisions that align with your values and individual needs.

BELIEF IN THE MIND-BODY CONNECTION

A fundamental pillar of cultivating faith in the healing process is recognizing and harnessing the power of the mind-body connection. Scientific research has increasingly shown that our thoughts, emotions, and beliefs can impact our physical health and well-being.

Positive thoughts and beliefs have been linked to improved treatment outcomes, reduced stress levels, enhanced immune function, and overall well-being. When we cultivate faith in the healing process, we create a positive mindset that promotes healing on a cellular level. By nurturing positive thoughts and maintaining a hopeful outlook, we create an internal environment conducive to recovery and resilience.

Remember, cultivating faith does not mean denying the realities of cancer or overlooking the importance of medical interventions. Rather, it is about harnessing the power of the mind and spirit to complement and enhance the healing process. By embracing faith, we open ourselves to the possibility of transformation, resilience, and profound healing.

THE POWER OF HOPE

Hope is a powerful force that can transform our perspective and experience of battling cancer. It is the belief that there is a possibility of a positive outcome, even in the face of adversity. Embracing the power of hope can have a profound impact in overcoming our fears and on our well-being and treatment outcomes.

Maintaining a sense of hope can enhance our quality of life and foster a positive mindset throughout our cancer journey. To embrace the power of hope, it is crucial to focus on the aspects of our lives that bring us joy and meaning. Engaging in activities that bring us happiness, surrounding ourselves with positive influences, and celebrating even the smallest victories can help nurture and strengthen our sense of hope.

Cultivating a positive mindset is closely intertwined with embracing hope. By consciously shifting our thoughts towards positivity and optimism, we can cultivate resilience and overcome challenges more effectively. Challenging negative thoughts and replacing them with positive affirmations can help reframe our perspective and instill a sense of hope.

Seeking support from our loved ones and healthcare team also plays a significant role in maintaining hope. Building a strong support network and surrounding ourselves with individuals who uplift and inspire us can provide the encouragement and reassurance needed during difficult times.

CULTIVATING RESILIENCE

Resilience is the ability to recover from adversity and adapt to difficult conditions or circumstances. When battling cancer, cultivating resilience is essential for maintaining emotional well-being and promoting a positive outlook. Resilience enables us to face setbacks, endure treatments, and embrace the journey with strength and determination.

Resilience is not about denying the challenges or suppressing emotions; it is about developing healthy coping mechanisms to navigate through difficult times. It involves harnessing inner resources, such as optimism, self-efficacy, and social support, to overcome obstacles and bounce back stronger.

PRACTICAL STRATEGIES FOR LETTING GO OF FEAR, CULTIVATING FAITH AND EMBRACING HOPE AND RESILIENCE

1. *Knowledge is Power.* Educate Yourself about Cancer—understanding the disease, its treatment options, and the potential outcomes can help alleviate fear and provide a sense of control. Seek reliable sources of information, ask questions, and involve yourself in decision-making processes related to your care.

2. *Embracing Self-Care.* Taking care of your physical, emotional, and mental well-being is vital in cultivating resilience. Engage in activities that bring you joy and relaxation, practice stress-reducing techniques like meditation or deep breathing exercises, and ensure you prioritize your health by getting enough rest and maintaining a balanced diet.

3. *Embracing Positivity.* Surround yourself with positive influences, whether it is uplifting books, inspiring stories, or supportive communities. Choose to focus on positive aspects of your life, such as gratitude, hope, and acts of kindness. Embracing positivity can help shift your mindset from fear to hope and resilience.

4. *Mindfulness and Meditation.* Engaging in mindfulness practices can help quiet the mind, reduce anxiety, and enhance trust in the present moment. Meditation allows us to tap into our inner wisdom, connect with our breath, and cultivate a sense of peace and calm amidst the storm of cancer treatment.

5. *Affirmations and Visualization.* Utilizing positive affirmations and visualization techniques can reframe negative thought patterns and reinforce faith in the healing process. By visualizing the body's cells vibrant and healthy, we send powerful messages to our subconscious mind, enhancing our belief in the body's innate healing abilities.

6. *Supportive Community.* Surrounding yourself with a supportive community of loved ones, fellow cancer survivors, or support groups can be immensely beneficial in fostering a sense of belonging and encouragement. Sharing experiences, fears, and triumphs with others who understand can provide emotional support, inspire hope, and strengthen faith in the healing process.

7. *Spirituality and Connection.* Engaging in spiritual practices or nurturing a sense of connection with something greater than ourselves can instill a deep sense of faith and purpose. Whether through prayer, meditation, or engaging in nature, these practices can provide solace, guidance, and a profound belief in the healing journey.

8. *Express Your Emotions.* It is important to allow yourself to express and process your emotions. Find healthy outlets for your feelings, such as journaling, talking to a therapist, or joining support groups. By acknowledging and exploring your emotions, you can release fear and make space for hope and resilience.

9. *Set Realistic Goals.* Setting small, achievable goals can provide a sense of purpose and progress. Focus on milestones that are within your control, such as maintaining a healthy lifestyle, engaging in activities you enjoy, and fostering meaningful relationships. Celebrate each accomplishment, no matter how small, as a step forward in your journey.

In the battle against cancer, letting go of fear, taming your inner critic and embracing faith, hope and resilience can make a significant difference in our overall well-being and treatment outcomes. Always remember that cancer does not define who you are. You have the power to shape your own narrative and choose how you respond to challenges. Embracing these values will empower you on your journey towards healing. Be gentle with yourself, practice self-compassion, and believe in your strength to overcome any obstacle that comes your way.

PART II

Harnessing the Mind's Healing Potential

5

CULTIVATING A HEALING MINDSET: HARNESSING THE POWER WITHIN

Cultivating a healing mindset is a transformative approach to health and well-being. Cultivating a healing mindset begins with embracing a positive outlook on life and nurturing positive thoughts and beliefs. It involves shifting our perspective and choosing to focus on possibilities rather than limitations. By adopting a positive mindset, we can tap into the body's natural healing abilities and create an environment conducive to recovery.

PRACTICAL STRATEGIES FOR CULTIVATING A HEALING MINDSET

1. *Practicing Gratitude.* Gratitude is a powerful tool that shifts our attention to the blessings and positive aspects of our lives. By regularly expressing gratitude for the things we appreciate, we foster a sense of contentment and create a foundation for a healing mindset.

2. *Positive Affirmations.* An affirmation is a positive statements that reinforce in one empowering beliefs. By consciously repeating affirmations that reflect our desired state of health and well-being, we can reprogram our subconscious mind and align our thoughts with our healing intentions.

3. *Engaging in Activities That Bring Joy.* Engaging in activities that bring us joy and fulfillment helps to nourish our mental and emotional well-being. Whether it is pursuing hobbies, spending time in nature, or connecting with loved ones, these

activities contribute to a positive mindset and enhance our overall sense of well-being.

4. *Self-Care Practices.* Taking care of our physical, emotional, and spiritual needs is an essential aspect of cultivating a healing mindset. Engaging in self-care practices such as regular exercise, proper nutrition, quality sleep, and stress management techniques supports our body's healing process and promotes overall well-being.

5. *Visualizing Health and Healing.* Visualization is a technique that involves creating vivid mental images of desired outcomes. By visualizing ourselves in a state of optimal health and imagining the healing process taking place within our bodies, we can reinforce positive beliefs and stimulate our body's healing mechanisms.

Through the cultivation of a positive outlook towards life, we create an environment that fosters healing and resilience. By integrating these practices into our lives and embracing a healing mindset, we empower ourselves to navigate the challenges of our healing journey with grace, optimism, and a renewed sense of purpose. Remember, within each of us lies the power to nurture our wellness from within.

THE POWER OF POSITIVE THINKING: SHAPING REALITY THROUGH PERCEPTION

Positive thinking is more than just having a cheerful disposition or wearing a smile on our faces. It is a mindset that involves consciously directing our thoughts, beliefs, and attitudes towards optimism, hope, and resilience. Positive thinking does not deny the challenges or difficulties we face; instead, it chooses to focus on the possibilities, solutions, and opportunities that lie within every situation.

Research has shown that positive thinking has a tangible impact on our physical health. A positive mindset has been associated with lower levels of stress, enhanced immune function, improved cardiovascular health, and a reduced risk of chronic diseases such as hypertension and diabetes. Moreover, positive thinking promotes faster recovery from illnesses and surgeries, as it supports the body's natural healing mechanisms.

Our perception of reality is influenced by the thoughts, beliefs, and attitudes we hold. What we choose to focus on and how we interpret our experiences shapes our reality. Positive thinking allows us to reframe challenges as opportunities for growth, setbacks as temporary hurdles, and failures as stepping stones towards success.

PRACTICAL STRATEGIES FOR CULTIVATING POSITIVE THINKING

Self-Awareness. The first step in cultivating positive thinking is developing self-awareness. Pay attention to your thoughts and notice any patterns of negative thinking or self-limiting beliefs. By becoming aware of these patterns, you can consciously choose to replace them with positive and empowering thoughts.

Positive Affirmations. An affirmation is a positive statement or declaration that reinforce desired beliefs and outcomes. Repeat affirmations that align with your goals and aspirations. For example, if you are facing a health challenge, repeat affirmations such as "I am strong, healthy, and capable of healing." Over time, these affirmations will become embedded in your subconscious mind, shaping your perception and reality.

Gratitude Practice. Cultivating gratitude is a powerful way to shift your focus towards positivity. Taking a few moments each day to reflect on the things you are grateful for has proven to be a helpful way to harness the power of an optimistic mind. This practice enhances your appreciation for the present moment and reminds you of the abundance in your life.

Surround Yourself with Positivity. Surrounding yourself with positive influences can significantly impact your thinking patterns. Seek out supportive friends, mentors, or communities that uplift and inspire you. Engage in activities that bring you joy and expose yourself to positive media and literature.

Visualize Success. Visualization is a powerful technique that involves creating mental images of your desired outcomes. Take time to visualize yourself achieving your goals, whether it's recovering from an illness, excelling in your career, or cultivating fulfilling relationships. By vividly imagining success, you enhance your belief in your ability to achieve it.

Challenge Negative Thoughts. When negative thoughts arise, consciously challenge them. Ask yourself if they are based on facts or if they are simply assumptions or self-limiting beliefs. Replace negative thoughts with positive and empowering alternatives.

6

VISUALIZATION TECHNIQUES: CREATING A HEALING INNER SANCTUARY

In the battle against cancer, harnessing the power of the mind is a vital component of the healing process. One powerful technique that can assist in this journey is visualization. Visualization is a powerful tool that allows us to tap into the mind's creative capacity and influence our physical and emotional well-being. It involves using the imagination to create vivid mental images that evoke positive emotions and sensations. It is a process of consciously directing our thoughts to create a desired outcome. By engaging all our senses, we can create a comprehensive mental experience that stimulates our mind and body.

Visualization is based on the principle that our minds cannot distinguish between a vividly imagined experience and reality. When we visualize ourselves in a state of health and well-being, our mind and body respond as if it were true. This phenomenon is supported by scientific research in the field of psychoneuroimmunology, which explores the connection between our thoughts, emotions, and our immune system.

Visualizing the healing process involves imagining your body's cells working harmoniously, eliminating cancerous cells, and restoring health and vitality—picturing your immune system as a strong and efficient defense mechanism, targeting and destroying cancer cells. Engaging in this practice regularly can promote a positive mindset and support your body's natural healing mechanisms.

Visualization can also be used to release emotions and reduce stress, which are crucial aspects of the healing journey. Through visualization, you can imagine releasing fear, anxiety, and any negative emotions associated with your cancer diagnosis. This process helps create an internal environment conducive to healing and supports emotional well-being.

Visualizing your desired outcomes and goals can provide clarity and motivation throughout your cancer journey. Whether it is visualizing the successful completion of treatment, returning to activities you love, or envisioning a future free from cancer, creating a mental image of your goals reinforces your determination and activates the subconscious mind to work towards those goals.

Like any skill, mastering visualization requires consistent practice. You ought to set aside dedicated time each day to engage in visualization exercises. Find a quiet space, close your eyes, and fully immerse yourself in the visualization process. The more you practice, the more effective your visualizations will become.

Remember, visualization should be used as a complementary practice alongside conventional medical treatments. It is not a replacement for medical advice or interventions. However, by incorporating visualization into your daily routine, you can cultivate a sense of empowerment, resilience, and hope as you navigate the challenges of battling cancer.

INTEGRATING VISUALIZATION INTO DAILY LIFE: PRACTICAL TECHNIQUES AND EXERCISES

1. *Guided Imagery.* Guided imagery, also known as guided visualization involves following a recorded script or the guidance of a trained professional. It is using the imagination to create vivid mental images that promote relaxation, well-being, and healing through following These scripts often include visualizing the body's cells as healthy and vibrant, imagining the successful outcome of medical treatments, and embracing feelings of peace, strength, and optimism. It provides a structured approach to visualization, making it accessible to beginners. Guided imagery often includes soothing music, relaxation techniques, and specific imagery designed to promote healing and well-being.

2. *Creating a Healing Sanctuary.* Imagine a serene and peaceful sanctuary within your mind where you can retreat to whenever you need a moment of calm and healing. Visualize this sanctuary in vivid detail, incorporating elements that bring you joy and a sense of peace. You can visualize the sights, sounds, scents, and sensations of this healing sanctuary, allowing yourself to feel fully immersed in its tranquility.

3. *Healing Light Visualization.* Visualize a warm and healing light surrounding your body. Imagine this light as a powerful force of healing energy, penetrating every cell and tissue. Visualize the light clearing away any illness or imbalance and replacing it with vibrant health and vitality. Allow yourself to bask in the warmth and healing power of this light, knowing that it is nourishing your body and supporting your healing journey.

4. *Future Self Visualization.* Imagine your future self, free from cancer and thriving in health. Visualize yourself engaging in activities you love, surrounded by loved ones, and living a vibrant life. Create a detailed mental image of your future self, incorporating all the aspects that contribute to your well-being. By visualizing your desired future, you are setting a powerful intention and creating a positive blueprint for your healing journey.

5. *Gratitude Visualization.* Take a few moments each day to visualize and express gratitude for the positive aspects of your life. Close your eyes and imagine all the things you are grateful for, focusing on the feelings of appreciation and joy that arise. By cultivating gratitude through visualization, you are shifting your focus towards the positive aspects of your life, fostering a sense of well-being, and enhancing your ability to navigate the challenges of cancer with a hopeful mindset.

Integrating these visualization techniques into your daily life can be a transformative practice on your cancer journey. By harnessing the power of your imagination and engaging in practical techniques and exercises, you can shape your reality and promote healing from within. Embrace the power of visualization as a tool to cultivate resilience, empower yourself, and support your overall well-being in the face of cancer.

HOW VISUALIZATION SUPPORTS HEALING

1. *Stress Reduction.* Cancer diagnosis and treatment can be accompanied by significant emotional and psychological stress. Visualization provides a safe space for individuals to

relax and let go of stress. By engaging the imagination and creating positive mental images, it helps shift the focus away from worries and fears, promoting a sense of calm and tranquility.

2. *Immune System Activation.* Visualization has been shown to have a positive impact on the immune system. As you visualize your body's cells working harmoniously and envision a state of vibrant health, your mind communicates this message to your immune system. This activation can strengthen the body's natural defenses and promote a healthy immune response.

3. *Pain Management.* Chronic pain is often associated with cancer and its treatments. Visualization can be used as a complementary technique to manage pain by redirecting focus and creating a mental environment that promotes relaxation and relief. By visualizing the pain dissipating or being replaced with sensations of comfort and ease, individuals can experience a reduction in pain intensity and an overall improvement in well-being.

4. *Enhancing Treatment Outcomes.* When used in conjunction with conventional cancer treatments, visualization can enhance treatment outcomes. Research suggests that patients who engage in guided imagery during chemotherapy or radiation therapy may experience reduced side effects such as nausea, fatigue, and anxiety. By creating positive mental images of the treatment working effectively, individuals can positively influence their experience and support the body's response to treatment.

5. *Emotional Support and Coping.* Dealing with cancer can evoke a range of complex emotions. Visualization provides a platform for emotional exploration and support. Through

this process, individuals can connect with their inner strength, cultivate resilience, and find solace in moments of uncertainty. It aids individuals process and release emotions, allowing for a greater sense of emotional well-being and improved coping strategies.

6. *Empowerment and Positive Mindset.* Visualization empowers individuals by allowing them to actively participate in their healing process. By painting a mental canvas of healing and envisioning a positive outcome, individuals cultivate a sense of hope and agency. This empowerment enhances the belief in one's ability to heal and promotes a positive mindset that is vital in battling cancer.

7. *Personalized and Tailored Experience.* Visualization can be personalized to individual preferences and needs. Whether it's visualizing specific aspects of the healing process, connecting with inner resources, or embracing specific qualities such as strength or courage, the practice can be tailored to meet individual goals and aspirations. This personalization allows for a deeply meaningful and impactful experience.

Incorporating guided imagery into your cancer journey can enhance your overall well-being, improve treatment outcomes, and foster a positive mindset. It is important to remember that guided imagery is a complementary technique that works alongside conventional medical treatments. Always consult with your healthcare provider and work with a trained professional to ensure that guided imagery is integrated safely and effectively into your care plan.

7

MEDITATION AND MINDFULNESS: FINDING STILLNESS ADMIST THE STORM

Another effective mind-healing practice that has gained significant attention in recent years is meditation. Meditation is a mind-body technique that involves training the mind to focus and redirect thoughts, resulting in a state of deep relaxation and heightened awareness.

Meditation is a practice that has been around for thousands of years and is rooted in ancient traditions. It involves sitting in a comfortable position, closing the eyes, and directing the attention inward. The goal of meditation is to achieve a state of mental clarity, emotional calmness, and inner peace. It is not about suppressing thoughts but rather observing them without judgment and allowing them to pass.

THE BENEFITS OF MEDITATION

1. *Stress Reduction.* Chronic stress can have a detrimental impact on physical and mental well-being. Meditation has been shown to activate the body's relaxation response, counteracting the effects of stress. By practicing meditation regularly, individuals can experience reduced stress levels, lower blood pressure, and improved overall well-being. This can be particularly beneficial for cancer patients, as managing stress is crucial during the treatment and recovery process.

2. *Immune System Support.* The immune system plays a vital role in fighting cancer and maintaining overall health. Research suggests that regular meditation can enhance

immune function by reducing inflammation, boosting the activity of natural killer cells, and promoting the production of antibodies. By calming the mind through meditation, individuals can support their immune system's ability to defend against cancer cells and promote healing.

3. *Pain Management.* Cancer and its treatments can often cause physical discomfort and pain. Meditation has been shown to reduce the perception of pain by activating areas in the brain associated with pain modulation and increasing the release of endorphins, the body's natural painkillers. By incorporating meditation into their routine, individuals battling cancer can experience relief from pain and a greater sense of well-being.

4. *Emotional Well-being.* Cancer can evoke a range of emotions, including fear, anxiety, and sadness. Meditation can be a powerful tool for managing these emotions by fostering emotional resilience and cultivating a sense of inner peace. Regular meditation practice can help individuals develop a greater sense of self-awareness, emotional balance, and compassion towards oneself and others, thus enhancing their emotional well-being during the cancer journey.

5. *Sleep Improvement.* Quality sleep is essential for overall health and healing. Cancer and its treatments can disrupt sleep patterns, leading to fatigue and compromised well-being. Meditation has been shown to improve sleep quality by calming the mind and reducing racing thoughts. By incorporating meditation into their daily routine, individuals can promote better sleep, enhance their energy levels, and support their body's healing processes.

PRACTICAL TECHNIQUES AND EXERCISES

1. *Mindfulness Meditation.* Mindfulness meditation is a popular form of meditation that involves paying attention to the present moment without judgment. It focuses on observing thoughts, sensations, and emotions as they arise, allowing individuals to cultivate a sense of mindfulness and self-awareness. By practicing mindfulness meditation, individuals can train their minds to stay present, reduce stress, and enhance overall well-being.

2. *Loving-Kindness Meditation.* Loving-kindness meditation involves directing well-wishes and compassion towards oneself and others. It cultivates feelings of love, empathy, and kindness, fostering a sense of connection and emotional well-being. By practicing loving-kindness meditation, individuals can enhance their ability to navigate the challenges of cancer with a compassionate and open heart.

3. *Body Scan Meditation.* Body scan meditation involves systematically directing attention to different parts of the body, observing physical sensations, and promoting relaxation. It can help individuals develop a deeper connection with their bodies, enhance body awareness, and alleviate tension and discomfort. By practicing body scan meditation, individuals can promote a sense of harmony between the mind and body, supporting the healing process.

By incorporating meditation into their daily lives, individuals can experience reduced stress, enhanced immune function, improved pain management, emotional well-being, and better sleep quality. Do not forget to consult with your healthcare provider to ensure that meditation practices are tailored to your specific needs and integrated safely into your cancer care plan. Embrace the power of meditation, and let it be a source of healing and strength on your cancer journey.

EMBRACING MINDFULNESS: BEING PRESENT IN THE MOMENT

Mindfulness is a practice that involves paying attention to the present moment with openness, curiosity, and non-judgment. It is the art of being fully present in the here and now, without being caught up in judgments or distractions. It involves intentionally directing our attention to the present moment, observing our thoughts, emotions, and sensations with an attitude of acceptance and non-reactivity. Mindfulness is not about emptying the mind or trying to suppress thoughts; rather, it is about cultivating awareness and compassion towards ourselves and our experiences.

THE BENEFITS OF MINDFULNESS

1. *Stress Reduction.* Cancer can bring about a myriad of stressors, including uncertainty, fear, and anxiety. Mindfulness has been shown to reduce stress by activating the body's relaxation response and decreasing the production of stress hormones. By practicing mindfulness, individuals can develop greater resilience and coping mechanisms, helping to alleviate the burden of stress associated with cancer.

2. *Emotional Well-being.* The emotional toll of cancer can be significant, impacting mood, self-esteem, and overall well-being. Mindfulness allows individuals to observe their thoughts and emotions without judgment, creating space for self-compassion and self-care. By embracing mindfulness, individuals can develop a more positive and accepting

relationship with themselves, fostering emotional well-being throughout their cancer journey.

3. *Pain Management.* Cancer and its treatments can often cause physical pain and discomfort. Mindfulness has been shown to reduce the perception of pain by shifting attention away from pain sensations and cultivating a non-judgmental awareness of the body. By incorporating mindfulness into their daily lives, individuals can develop a greater ability to manage pain and enhance their overall quality of life.

4. *Improved Cognitive Function.* Cancer and its treatments can sometimes impact cognitive function, leading to difficulties with concentration, memory, and decision-making. Mindfulness practices, such as focused attention and open monitoring, have been found to enhance cognitive abilities, including attention, working memory, and cognitive flexibility. By embracing mindfulness, individuals can sharpen their mental focus and enhance cognitive function.

5. *Enhanced Quality of Life.* Mindfulness offers a pathway to finding joy and meaning in life, even in the face of adversity. By being fully present and engaged in each moment, individuals can savor the simple pleasures, foster gratitude, and cultivate a deeper sense of connection with themselves and others. By embracing mindfulness, individuals can enhance their overall quality of life, finding moments of peace and joy amidst the challenges of cancer.

TECHNIQUES FOR CULTIVATING MINDFULNESS

1. *Mindful Breathing.* One of the simplest and most accessible ways to practice mindfulness is through mindful breathing. Take a few moments each day to focus your attention on the sensation of your breath as it enters and leaves your body.

Notice the rise and fall of your abdomen or the sensation of air passing through your nostrils. Whenever your mind wanders, gently bring your focus back to the breath, anchoring yourself in the present moment.

2. *The Body Scan Technique.* The body scan is a practice that involves systematically directing attention to different parts of the body, observing sensations without judgment. Starting from the top of your head and moving down to your toes, bring your awareness to each body part, noticing any sensations or areas of tension. Allow yourself to fully experience the sensations, acknowledging them with an attitude of curiosity and acceptance.

3. *Mindful Eating.* Eating mindfully involves savoring each bite of food with full awareness. Slow down and pay attention to the taste, texture, and aroma of your food. Notice the sensations in your mouth and the act of chewing. Engage your senses fully, appreciating the nourishment and pleasure that food brings. By practicing mindful eating, you can develop a healthier relationship with food and cultivate a sense of gratitude for nourishing your body.

INCORPORATING MEDITATION INTO YOUR DAILY LIFE

1. *Create a Sacred Space.* Designate a quiet and peaceful space in your home where you can practice meditation without distractions. Make it a comfortable and inviting space with soft lighting, cushions, or a meditation chair. This space will serve as a sanctuary for your practice, allowing you to fully immerse yourself in the meditation experience.

2. *Set a Regular Practice Time.* Establish a regular meditation routine by choosing a specific time of day that works best for you. It can be in the morning, before bed, or during a quiet moment in the afternoon. Consistency is key in reaping the benefits of meditation, so aim to meditate for a few minutes each day and gradually increase the duration as you feel comfortable.

3. *Start with Short Sessions.* If you're new to meditation, begin with shorter sessions, such as five to ten minutes, and gradually increase the duration over time. This will allow you to build your meditation practice gradually and avoid feeling overwhelmed or discouraged.

4. *Seek Guidance.* Consider seeking guidance from a meditation teacher, mindfulness instructor, or joining a meditation group or class. They can provide valuable guidance, support, and help tailor meditation practices to your specific needs and circumstances. Working with a professional can also help you address any challenges or questions that may arise during your meditation journey.

5. *Integrate Meditation into Daily Activities.* In addition to formal meditation sessions, look for opportunities to integrate mindfulness into your daily activities. Practice mindful eating by savoring each bite of food, engage in mindful walking by paying attention to your steps and the sensations in your body, or practice mindful listening by fully focusing on the sounds around you. These small moments of mindfulness can bring greater awareness and presence to your day.

6. *Follow a Step-by-Step Process.* Here is a step-by-step process to guide you through a basic meditation session:

a. Find a comfortable seated position with an upright posture.

b. Close your eyes or maintain a soft gaze, whichever feels comfortable for you.

c. Bring your attention to your breath, noticing the sensation of each inhalation and exhalation.

d. As thoughts arise, gently acknowledge them without judgment and redirect your focus back to the breath.

e. Continue to observe your breath and any sensations, thoughts, or emotions that arise, allowing them to come and go without attachment.

f. If you find your mind wandering, gently bring your attention back to the breath.

g. As your session comes to a close, take a few deep breaths and slowly open your eyes.

7. *Practice Regularly.* Consistency is the key to reaping the benefits of meditation and mindfulness. Aim to practice meditation daily, even if it's for a few minutes. Gradually increase the duration of your sessions as you become more comfortable and committed to your practice.

Meditation is a transformative practice that can empower you on your journey towards better health and well-being. Remember, meditation is a personal journey, and it may take time to find the techniques and practices that resonate with you. Be patient, be kind to yourself, and enjoy the process of deepening your meditation practice.

8

THE HEALING INFLUENCE OF EMOTIONAL WELL-BEING

Emotional well-being encompasses a wide range of aspects, including our thoughts, feelings, and attitudes towards ourselves and the world around us. It is the state of being in tune with our emotions, recognizing them, and responding to them in a healthy and balanced way. When it comes to cancer, cultivating emotional well-being is not about finding a quick fix or dismissing the reality of the disease. Instead, it is about harnessing the inherent power within ourselves to navigate the challenges, find inner strength, and optimize our overall well-being.

Cancer is not just a physical battle; it is also an emotional and mental challenge. Nurturing emotional well-being empowers us to face the diagnosis with resilience, courage, and a positive mindset. It allows us to tap into our inner resources, build a sense of control, and develop coping strategies that can positively influence our healing journey.

Emotional well-being can enhance the effectiveness of medical treatments. Research suggests that individuals with a positive mindset and emotional well-being may experience better treatment outcomes, improved tolerance of side effects, and increased adherence to treatment plans. By fostering emotional well-being, we create a fertile ground for our body to respond optimally to the treatments we receive.

Emotional well-being is not solely an individual pursuit. It also involves nurturing social connections and seeking support from loved ones, support groups, or counseling services. These connections provide a supportive network and a safe space to express emotions, share experiences, and receive encouragement during the cancer journey.

In the pages that follow, we will explore various strategies, techniques, and practices to cultivate emotional well-being and harness its healing influence. Together, we will embark on a transformative journey that empowers you to tap into the power of your mind and emotions, creating a foundation for healing and a renewed sense of vitality in your life.

HEALING EMOTIONAL WOUNDS: ADDRESSING PAST TRAUMA

In the battle against cancer, the power of the mind extends far beyond positive thinking and emotional well-being. It also involves addressing the emotional wounds and traumas that may have shaped our lives. Unresolved past traumas can have a profound impact on our physical health, including our ability to cope with and heal from cancer.

Emotional wounds, such as childhood trauma, loss, abuse, or significant life challenges, can create deep-seated emotional pain and distress. These wounds are not confined to the past; they continue to influence our thoughts, emotions, and behaviors in the present. When facing cancer, these unresolved emotional wounds can manifest as stress, anxiety, depression, and can even hinder the body's ability to heal. By addressing and healing these emotional wounds, we can positively impact our body's ability to heal and enhance our overall well-being.

The first step in healing emotional wounds is to uncover and acknowledge their existence. This requires self-reflection, courage, and a willingness to explore our past experiences. It may be helpful to seek the support of a therapist or counselor who specializes in trauma therapy. They can provide a safe and supportive environment to navigate the complexities of past trauma and guide you towards healing.

Once emotional wounds are identified, the healing process involves processing and releasing the emotional pain associated with them. This may involve various therapeutic modalities such as cognitive-behavioral therapy, Eye Movement Desensitization and Reprocessing (EMDR), somatic experiencing, or expressive arts therapy. These techniques facilitate the release of stored emotions and help rewire the brain's response to trauma, paving the way for healing and growth.

As we heal from emotional wounds, it is also essential to develop healthy coping strategies to manage the emotional challenges that may arise during the cancer journey. This can include mindfulness practices, deep breathing exercises, journaling, or engaging in creative outlets such as painting or writing. These strategies provide a constructive outlet for emotions, promote self-care, and foster resilience.

Healing emotional wounds is not a linear process, and it requires patience and self-compassion. It is essential to surround yourself with a supportive network of loved ones, participate in support groups, and seek professional guidance when needed. These resources provide emotional support, validation, and encouragement as you navigate the healing journey.

THE IMPACT ON CANCER TREATMENT

Addressing past trauma and healing emotional wounds can have a profound impact on the effectiveness of cancer treatment. By releasing emotional distress, reducing stress levels, and promoting emotional well-being, the body's natural healing mechanisms are enhanced, and treatment outcomes may be improved. Additionally, healing emotional wounds can positively influence treatment adherence, decision-making, and overall quality of life.

Healing emotional wounds allows us to create a new narrative for ourselves, one that is free from the constraints of past trauma. It opens the door to personal growth, self-empowerment, and a renewed sense of purpose. By embracing our capacity to heal emotionally, we can shape a more resilient mindset that supports our physical and emotional well-being throughout the cancer journey.

Addressing past trauma and healing emotional wounds is a vital component of harnessing the power of the mind in battling cancer. By acknowledging and processing these wounds, we can pave the way for emotional well-being, resilience, and enhanced healing. The journey may be challenging, but with the right support and a commitment to self-care, we can embark on a transformative path towards holistic healing and renewed vitality.

NURTURING RELATIONSHIPS: CULTIVATING A SUPPORTIVE NETWORK

Additionally, our relationships and the support we receive from our loved ones play a vital role in shaping our emotional well-being and overall ability to cope with the challenges of cancer. Social support refers to the network of relationships and connections we have with others. It encompasses emotional, practical, and informational support provided by family, friends, and the broader community.

Emotional Support. Emotional support is a cornerstone of nurturing relationships. It involves receiving understanding, empathy, and compassion from others, which can help alleviate stress, anxiety, and feelings of isolation. Sharing fears, concerns, and emotions with trusted individuals creates a sense of validation and comfort, fostering a positive mindset and emotional resilience.

Practical Support. Practical support encompasses the tangible assistance that others can provide during the cancer journey. This may include help with transportation to medical appointments, cooking meals, running errands, or providing childcare. By relieving some of the burdens and responsibilities, practical support allows individuals to focus on their well-being, treatment, and recovery.

Informational Support. Informational support involves the provision of relevant and accurate information about cancer, treatment options, and available resources. It helps individuals make informed decisions and empowers them to actively participate in their treatment journey. Access to reliable information can alleviate anxiety and promote a sense of control and confidence.

BUILDING BONDS AND STRENGTHENING RELATIONSHIPS

Cultivating a supportive network requires effort and open communication. Here are some strategies to build and strengthen relationships during the cancer journey:

1. *Communication.* Openly express your needs, fears, and concerns to your loved ones. Clear communication fosters understanding and allows others to provide meaningful support.

2. *Seek Understanding.* Encourage your loved ones to learn about cancer and its impact. This promotes empathy, reduces misconceptions, and facilitates a supportive environment.

3. *Boundaries.* Set boundaries and communicate your limits. It is okay to ask for privacy or specify the type of support you require. Respectful boundaries promote healthier and more sustainable relationships.

4. *Join Support Groups.* Participate in cancer support groups where you can connect with others who understand your experience. Sharing stories, advice, and encouragement can be immensely comforting.

5. *Express Gratitude.* Show appreciation for the support you receive. A simple thank you, handwritten note, or small gesture can go a long way in nurturing relationships and maintaining strong bonds.

THE RECIPROCAL NATURE OF SUPPORT

While it is essential to receive support, it is equally important to offer support to others. Engaging in acts of kindness and providing support to those in need fosters a sense of purpose and belonging. By contributing to the well-being of others, we reinforce the positive energy within our own lives.

In addition to the support of family and friends, seeking professional support can be immensely beneficial. Psychologists, counselors, and support services specializing in cancer care can provide a safe and confidential space to address emotional concerns, offer guidance, and develop coping strategies tailored to your specific needs.

It is also important to acknowledge that relationships may face challenges during the cancer journey. Loved ones may struggle with their own emotions, fears, or difficulties in providing the support you need. It is crucial to communicate openly, express your feelings, and seek professional help if necessary. Remember that these challenges can be an opportunity for growth and deeper connection when addressed with empathy and understanding.

Nurturing relationships and cultivating a supportive network are essential components of harnessing the power of the mind in battling cancer. By building and strengthening relationships, expressing gratitude, and seeking professional support, individuals can create a network of support that empowers them to navigate the challenges of cancer with resilience, hope, and a positive mindset.

THE ROLE OF GRATITUDE AND FORGIVENESS: EMBRACING JOY AND LETTING GO

Gratitude is a powerful practice that involves consciously focusing on the positive aspects of life, even in the midst of adversity. When facing cancer, it can be easy to get caught up in fear, pain, and uncertainty. However, cultivating gratitude allows us to shift our perspective and acknowledge the blessings that still exist. By directing our attention to the things we are grateful for, we invite more positivity and joy into our lives.

Practicing gratitude is not about denying or minimizing the challenges of cancer, but rather about finding moments of beauty, love, and connection amidst the hardships. It could be appreciating the support of loved ones, the kindness of strangers, the beauty of nature, or the small victories along the treatment journey. By actively seeking out and acknowledging these blessings, we cultivate a sense of abundance and optimism that can uplift our spirits and contribute to our overall well-being.

Forgiveness is also a powerful tool for emotional healing and personal growth. Holding onto anger, resentment, or bitterness can create emotional toxicity, which can impact our physical health and well-being. Forgiveness is not about condoning or forgetting past wrongs; rather, it is a choice to release the negative emotions associated with those experiences and free ourselves from their grip.

When we forgive, we let go of the burden of carrying anger and resentment. It is an act of self-compassion and liberation. By releasing negative emotions, we create space for love, joy, and healing to enter our lives. Forgiveness allows us to move forward with a lighter heart and a renewed sense of purpose.

Gratitude and forgiveness, which are crucial steps towards embracing joy, are powerful practices that can transform our experience of battling cancer. By cultivating gratitude, we shift our focus to the blessings in our lives, fostering a sense of abundance and optimism. Forgiveness liberates us from the weight of anger and resentment, creating space for healing and growth. Embracing these values allows us to experience the richness of life, even in the face of challenges.

Moreover, gratitude and forgiveness has been linked to improved mental and physical health outcomes. Medical research has shown that individuals who practice them experience reduced levels of stress, anxiety, and depression. They also report higher levels of life satisfaction, improved immune function, and better cardiovascular health.

9

EMBRACING THE GIFTS OF CANCER: TRANSFORMING ADVERSITY INTO OPPORTUNITY

From the title of this chapter, it may seem counterintuitive to think of cancer, one of the most horrendous words in the medical world, as a gift. You may even go further to question why I would term it so. However, in this chapter we aim at exploring the concept of embracing the gifts of cancer and how it can empower individuals to transform adversity into opportunity.

One of the gifts that cancer can bring is an opportunity to reflect on our lives and reassess our priorities. It prompts us to question our values, goals, and the way we have been living. Through this introspection, we can discover a renewed sense of purpose and meaning. Cancer becomes a catalyst for transformation, inspiring us to make positive changes in our lives and pursue what truly matters to us.

Cancer can also gift us with a deeper sense of connection and support. It often brings people together – family, friends, and even strangers – who provide love, care, and encouragement during our journey. It is an opportunity to witness the incredible power of human compassion and experience the strength of community. By embracing these connections and allowing ourselves to receive support, we create a network that uplifts and sustains us throughout the healing process.

While cancer presents immense challenges, it also offers a platform for personal growth and the development of resilience. Through the trials and tribulations of treatment, we discover strengths we never knew we had. We learn to navigate uncertainty, face our fears, and persevere in the face of adversity. The challenges of cancer push us to tap into our inner resilience, helping us emerge as stronger individuals.

Cancer provides an opportunity for deep self-reflection and self-care. It compels us to prioritize our well-being and engage in practices that nurture our physical, emotional, and spiritual health. It encourages us to listen to our bodies, practice self-compassion, and make choices that promote healing and balance. Through self-reflection and self-care, we cultivate a strong foundation for our overall well-being.

For many, the journey with cancer can be a catalyst for spiritual awakening and transcendence. It invites us to explore our beliefs, connect with our inner spirituality, and seek a deeper understanding of life's mysteries. Cancer can ignite a profound spiritual transformation, allowing us to tap into inner reserves of strength, find solace in faith, and experience a sense of connection to something greater than ourselves.

Finally, the gifts of cancer empower individuals to make a difference in the lives of others. It inspires us to become advocates, support networks, and sources of hope for those who are also battling cancer. By sharing our experiences, insights, and lessons learned, we become a beacon of light and inspiration for others on their own journey.

SHIFTING PERSPECTIVES: FINDING SILVER LININGS IN THE CANCER JOURNEY

In the midst of a cancer diagnosis, it can be challenging to see beyond the darkness and uncertainty. Here the power of the mind becomes very crucial. By harnessing the power of the mind, individuals can cultivate a positive outlook, embrace resilience, and discover hidden blessings amidst the challenges of battling cancer.

Our perception shapes our reality, and it plays a crucial role in how we experience and navigate the cancer journey. Shifting our perspective involves consciously choosing to see beyond the difficulties and focusing on the opportunities for growth, learning, and transformation. By reframing our thoughts and beliefs, we can cultivate a mindset that empowers us to find silver linings even in the face of adversity.

Cancer tests our physical and emotional strength, but it also reveals the depths of our inner resilience. By shifting our perspective, we can recognize the inner strength that lies within us. It allows us to tap into our innate courage, determination, and perseverance. Through the challenges of the cancer journey, we unearth a newfound sense of empowerment and discover our ability to overcome obstacles.

While cancer can feel isolating, it also has the power to foster deep connections with others. As such, we ought to recognize the opportunity to build meaningful relationships and receive support from loved ones, healthcare professionals, and support networks. Through shared experiences and mutual support, we can find solace, strength, and a sense of belonging.

Shifting perspectives can also open doors to new opportunities and possibilities. Cancer may redirect our life paths, encouraging us to explore new passions, hobbies, or career aspirations. Thus, by embracing change and allowing ourselves to grow and evolve, we can uncover hidden talents, explore new interests, and find fulfillment in unexpected ways.

Shifting perspectives and finding silver linings in the cancer journey is a transformative practice that empowers individuals to navigate the challenges with strength, resilience, and grace. By consciously choosing to see beyond the difficulties, we can unlock the hidden blessings within the cancer journey. This shift in perspective not only enhances our own well-being but also inspires and uplifts those around us, creating a ripple effect of positivity and hope in the face of adversity.

THE CALL TO AUTHENTICITY: ALIGNING LIFE WITH VALUES AND PASSIONS

Through the cancer journey, individuals often experience a deep reflection on their lives and priorities. The call to authenticity emerges as a powerful force, urging individuals to align their lives with their core values and passions.

Authenticity is the state of being true to oneself, living in alignment with one's core values, beliefs, and passions. It involves embracing and expressing one's unique identity, rather than conforming to societal expectations or external pressures. In the context of cancer, the call to authenticity becomes even more pronounced, as individuals are confronted with the fragility of life and the importance of living in accordance with their true selves.

Cancer serves as a catalyst for self-reflection, prompting individuals to reevaluate their priorities and align their lives with their core values. By identifying and embracing these fundamental principles, individuals can make choices that honor their true selves, fostering a sense of purpose, meaning, and fulfillment. Living in alignment with core values empowers individuals to make decisions that support their overall well-being and enhances their ability to navigate the challenges of the cancer journey.

The cancer journey also provides an opportunity for individuals to reconnect with their passions and creativity. By answering the call to authenticity, individuals can tap into their inner reservoirs of inspiration and pursue activities that bring joy and fulfillment. Engaging in creative endeavors, such as art, music, writing, or any other form of self-expression, can be therapeutic and provide a sense of empowerment and liberation during the healing process.

Authenticity further invites individuals to express themselves fully, embracing their true thoughts, emotions, and desires. Cancer can sometimes lead to feelings of vulnerability, fear, and uncertainty. However, by embracing self-expression, individuals can find solace and release. This can be achieved through journaling, talking with loved ones, participating in support groups, or seeking the guidance of a professional therapist. Authentic self-expression enables individuals to navigate the emotional complexities of the cancer journey and foster emotional well-being.

Living authentically often requires creating a supportive environment that honors one's true self. This may involve setting boundaries, communicating needs and desires, and surrounding oneself with individuals who support and uplift. By cultivating a network of understanding and compassionate individuals, individuals can draw strength, encouragement, and inspiration. Authenticity thrives in an environment that fosters acceptance, understanding, and encouragement.

Embracing authenticity requires transcending the fear of judgment and societal expectations. Cancer can evoke feelings of self-doubt and vulnerability, but by embracing authenticity, individuals can find the strength to rise above external pressures and live according to their own truth. This liberation from the fear of judgment empowers individuals to make choices that align with their values and passions, fostering a sense of empowerment and inner peace.

Authenticity calls us to embrace the present moment fully. Cancer often heightens awareness of the preciousness of each day. By practicing mindfulness and being fully present, individuals can savor the simple joys and experiences that unfold. Embracing the present moment enhances well-being, reduces stress, and allows individuals to fully engage with life, even in the face of challenges.

Embracing authenticity is a courageous and transformative journey, particularly in the context of battling cancer. By aligning life with core values and passions, expressing oneself authentically, creating a supportive environment, transcending fear and judgment, and living fully in the present moment, individuals can unlock their true potential, find renewed purpose, and navigate the cancer journey with strength and resilience. The call to authenticity is a powerful invitation to embrace one's uniqueness, to live a life of meaning and fulfillment, and to find profound healing and empowerment in the face of adversity.

PART III

Empowering the Healing Journey

10

NUTRITIONAL HEALING: FUELING THE BODY FOR RECOVERY

In the cancer battle, it is very important to remember that the mind is not the only ally in this fight. Our bodies also play a crucial role, and one of the most powerful tools at our disposal is proper nutrition.

Nutrition is more than just fuel for the body. It plays a multifaceted role in both preventing and managing the disease. A well-balanced diet plays the very important role of strengthening the immune system, supporting healthy cell function, reducing inflammation, and providing the body with the essential nutrients needed for optimal health and recovery. By nourishing the body with the right foods, individuals can create an internal environment that is less conducive to cancer growth and more supportive of healing.

The food we consume has a profound impact on our overall health and well-being. In the context of cancer, making conscious and informed food choices becomes even more critical. Nutrient-dense foods, such as fresh fruits and vegetables, whole grains, lean proteins, and healthy fats, provide the body with the necessary building blocks for repair, regeneration, and immune function. Conversely, a diet high in processed foods, sugary beverages, and unhealthy fats can contribute to inflammation, oxidative stress, and a compromised immune system.

The immune system plays a vital role in recognizing and eliminating cancer cells. Proper nutrition is essential for maintaining a robust immune system. Certain nutrients, such as vitamin C, vitamin D, zinc, and antioxidants, have been shown to support immune function and help the body fight against cancer. By consuming a varied and nutrient-rich diet, individuals can give their immune system the support it needs to battle cancer cells and aid in the recovery process.

Cancer treatments such as chemotherapy, radiation, and surgery can often cause unwanted side effects that impact an individual's quality of life. Proper nutrition also helps in managing these side effects and support overall well-being during treatment. For example, consuming small, frequent meals can alleviate nausea and maintain energy levels, while increasing fluid and fiber intake can help alleviate constipation commonly associated with certain medications. By working with healthcare professionals and incorporating a targeted nutrition plan, individuals can effectively manage treatment-related side effects and support their recovery journey.

Lastly, it is important to note that nutrition is not a one-size-fits-all approach. Each person's nutritional needs may vary based on their individual health status, type of cancer, treatment plan, and other factors. Working with a healthcare team, including registered dietitians or nutritionists, can provide individuals with personalized guidance and support in developing a nutrition plan that suits their specific needs and goals.

Nutritional healing is a powerful complement to the power of the mind in battling cancer. Making conscious and informed food choices is an empowering step in the cancer journey, giving individuals a sense of control and actively contributing to their recovery process.

THE HEALING POWER OF FOOD

The foods we consume have a direct impact on our overall health and vitality. When it comes to cancer, understanding the nutritional landscape becomes even more critical. Cancer treatments can take a toll on the body, leading to side effects such as nausea, fatigue, and loss of appetite. Nourishing our bodies with the right foods can help mitigate these side effects, support immune function, and aid in the recovery process.

A well-balanced diet is essential for overall health. Nutrient-dense foods provide the body with a wide array of vitamins, minerals, antioxidants, and phytochemicals that support cellular function, boost the immune system, and promote overall well-being. Fresh fruits and vegetables, whole grains, lean proteins, and healthy fats form the foundation of a nutrient-rich diet that can help fortify the body in its fight against cancer.

1. *Antioxidants and Phytochemicals.* Antioxidants and phytochemicals are powerful compounds found in plant-based foods that have been extensively studied for their potential cancer-fighting properties. These compounds help neutralize harmful free radicals, reduce inflammation, and support cellular health. Colorful fruits and vegetables such as berries, leafy greens, cruciferous vegetables, and citrus fruits are excellent sources of antioxidants and phytochemicals. By

incorporating these foods into our diet, we can provide our bodies with the tools they need to combat cancer.

2. *Healthy Fats and Omega-3 Fatty Acids.* Healthy fats, particularly those rich in omega-3 fatty acids, play a crucial role in our overall health. Omega-3 fatty acids have been shown to possess anti-inflammatory properties and may help reduce the risk of certain types of cancer. Foods such as fatty fish (salmon, mackerel, sardines), walnuts, flaxseeds, and chia seeds are excellent sources of omega-3 fatty acids. Including these foods in our diet can contribute to a healthy inflammatory response and support our body's healing process.

3. *Fiber.* Fiber is an often-overlooked component of a healthy diet, but it plays a significant role in our digestive health and overall well-being. A high-fiber diet promotes regular bowel movements, helps maintain a healthy weight, and supports the growth of beneficial gut bacteria. Whole grains, legumes, fruits, vegetables, and nuts and seeds are all excellent sources of dietary fiber. By incorporating fiber-rich foods into our meals, we can support our digestive system and enhance our body's ability to absorb vital nutrients.

4. *Hydration and the Importance of Water.* Staying hydrated is essential for optimal health, especially during cancer treatment. Adequate hydration supports numerous bodily functions, including digestion, circulation, and detoxification. Water helps transport nutrients throughout the body and aids in the elimination of waste products. It is important to prioritize hydration and drink sufficient water throughout the day, even if the treatment may temporarily affect our sense of taste or appetite.

The healing power of food cannot be underestimated in the battle against cancer. Nutritional choices have the potential to support our bodies, enhance immune function, mitigate side effects of treatment, and contribute to overall well-being. Remember, every bite we take is an opportunity to nourish our bodies and support our healing journey.

AN ANTI-CANCER DIET: NUTRITIONAL
STRATEGIES FOR SUPPORT

While there is no magic food that can cure cancer, adopting an anti-cancer diet can provide our bodies with the necessary nutrients and support to strengthen our immune system, enhance treatment outcomes, and promote overall wellness.

An anti-cancer diet focuses on nourishing our bodies with nutrient-rich foods that have been shown to possess cancer-fighting properties. It is important to note that an anti-cancer diet should be seen as a complementary approach to conventional cancer treatments, not a substitute. Based on this, here are some recommendations for planning your diet:

1. *Emphasizing Plant-Based Foods.* Plant-based foods form the foundation of an anti-cancer diet. Fruits, vegetables, whole grains, legumes, nuts, and seeds are rich sources of vitamins, minerals, antioxidants, and phytochemicals that promote optimal health. These foods provide a diverse array of nutrients and bioactive compounds that have been associated with a reduced risk of various types of cancer. Aim to fill at least two-thirds of your plate with colorful fruits and vegetables to maximize their benefits.

2. *Cruciferous Vegetables.* Cruciferous vegetables, such as broccoli, cauliflower, kale, and Brussels sprouts, are particularly notable for their cancer-fighting properties. They contain a compound called sulforaphane, which has been shown to inhibit the growth of cancer cells and stimulate the body's detoxification processes. Including cruciferous vegetables in your diet can provide a significant boost to your anti-cancer efforts.

3. *Colorful Fruits and Berries.* Colorful fruits and berries are rich in antioxidants, vitamins, and phytochemicals that protect our cells from damage and inflammation. Blueberries, strawberries, raspberries, and cherries are particularly potent in their cancer-fighting properties. These fruits are not only delicious but also contribute to a healthy immune system and support the body's natural defenses against cancer.

4. *Whole Grains and Legumes.* Whole grains, such as brown rice, quinoa, whole wheat bread, and oats, are excellent sources of fiber, vitamins, and minerals. Fiber plays a crucial role in maintaining a healthy digestive system and supports the elimination of toxins from the body. Legumes, including beans, lentils, and chickpeas, are also rich in fiber and provide plant-based protein. Incorporating whole grains and legumes into your diet can help reduce the risk of certain cancers and support overall well-being.

5. *Healthy Fats and Omega-3s.* Including healthy fats in your anti-cancer diet is essential. Avocados, olive oil, nuts, and seeds are excellent sources of monounsaturated and polyunsaturated fats, including omega-3 fatty acids. Omega-3s have been associated with reduced inflammation and may help decrease the risk of certain types of cancer. These healthy fats also aid in the absorption of fat-soluble vitamins and support overall heart health.

6. *Protein Choices.* When it comes to protein, opt for lean sources such as poultry, fish, tofu, and legumes. These protein-rich foods provide essential amino acids necessary for cellular repair and immune function. Avoid processed meats, as they have been linked to an increased risk of cancer. If you choose to consume animal products, prioritize quality and opt

for organic, hormone-free, and grass-fed options when possible.

7. *Limiting Processed and Red Meats.* Processed meats, including bacon, sausage, hot dogs, and deli meats, have been classified as carcinogens by the World Health Organization. Red meats, such as beef, pork, and lamb, should be consumed in moderation. When consuming red meat, choose lean cuts and limit consumption to a few times per month. Instead, focus on incorporating plant-based proteins and seafood into your anti-cancer diet.

8. *Hydration and Healthy Beverages.* Staying hydrated is vital for overall health, especially during cancer treatment. Water should be your primary beverage of choice, aiming for at least eight cups per day. Herbal teas, such as green tea and chamomile tea, provide additional hydration and contain beneficial compounds that may support the body's defense against cancer. Limit sugary drinks, sodas, and excessive caffeine, as they can contribute to inflammation and disrupt overall health.

While nutrition is a key component of an anti-cancer diet, it is essential to acknowledge the importance of other lifestyle factors in battling cancer. Regular physical activity, stress management, adequate sleep, and avoiding tobacco and excessive alcohol consumption all contribute to overall health and well-being. Combining this nutritional approach with a healthy lifestyle, results in enhancing your body's resilience and overall well-being. Remember, every food choice you make is an opportunity to nourish your body and make a positive impact on your cancer journey.

NAVIGATING DIETARY CHALLENGES: PRACTICAL TIPS AND RECIPES

The cancer journey can be filled with dietary challenges, such as loss of appetite, taste changes, and digestive issues. Let's explore practical tips and recipes to help you navigate these challenges and ensure that you continue to receive the vital nutrients your body needs to fight cancer and support your overall well-being.

1. *Managing Loss of Appetite.* Cancer treatments and medications can sometimes lead to a loss of appetite, making it difficult to consume enough calories and nutrients. Here are some tips to manage this challenge:

a. Opt for smaller, frequent meals: Instead of three large meals, try eating five or six smaller meals throughout the day to make it more manageable and appealing.

b. Focus on nutrient-dense foods: Choose foods that pack a nutritional punch, such as avocados, nut butters, yogurt, and smoothies. These foods provide essential nutrients even in smaller quantities.

c. Experiment with flavors and textures: Play with different flavors and textures to stimulate your appetite. Try adding herbs, spices, and marinades to enhance the taste of your meals. You can also experiment with different cooking methods, such as grilling or roasting, to add variety to your meals.

2. *Dealing with Taste Changes.* Cancer treatments can sometimes cause changes in taste, making previously enjoyable foods taste different or unappealing. Here are some strategies to cope with taste changes:

a. Experiment with seasonings: Experiment with different seasonings, herbs, and spices to add flavor to your meals. Tangy flavors from citrus fruits or vinegar can help mask unpleasant tastes.

b. Serve food at room temperature: Some people find that serving food at room temperature reduces the intensity of certain tastes. Cold or hot foods can sometimes have stronger flavors.

c. Try new foods: While some foods may taste different, you may discover new foods that are more appealing. Be open to trying new fruits, vegetables, and proteins to find ones that you enjoy.

3. *Addressing Digestive Issues.* Digestive issues, such as nausea, vomiting, or diarrhea, can make it challenging to maintain a healthy diet. Here are some tips to manage these symptoms:

a. Eat smaller, frequent meals: Eating smaller meals throughout the day can help prevent overloading your digestive system and ease symptoms.

b. Stay hydrated: Sip on water, herbal teas, and clear broths to stay hydrated and support your digestive system. Avoid drinking large amounts of fluids during meals, as it can contribute to feelings of fullness and discomfort.

c. Choose easily digestible foods: Opt for easily digestible foods, such as cooked vegetables, lean proteins, and whole grains like rice or quinoa. Avoid spicy, greasy, or fried foods that may aggravate your digestive system.

4. *Maintaining Proper Hydration.* Proper hydration is essential for overall health and well-being, especially during cancer treatment. Here are some tips to ensure you stay hydrated:

a. Drink water throughout the day: Sip on water at regular intervals throughout the day to stay hydrated. Set a reminder if needed.

b. Include hydrating foods: Incorporate foods with high water content into your diet, such as watermelon, cucumbers, soups, and smoothies.

c. Limit caffeine and alcohol: Caffeinated and alcoholic beverages can contribute to dehydration. Limit your intake and opt for water, herbal teas, or infused water instead.

5. *Nutrient-Rich Recipes*. Here are a few nutrient-rich recipe ideas that are easy to prepare and packed with essential nutrients:

a. *Green Smoothie*. Blend together spinach, kale, banana, almond milk, and a scoop of protein powder for a nutrient-packed smoothie.

b. *Quinoa Salad*. Cook quinoa and mix it with diced vegetables, such as bell peppers, cucumbers, and cherry tomatoes. Add lemon juice, olive oil, and herbs for flavor.

c. *Oven-Roasted Salmon*. Season salmon fillets with herbs, lemon juice, and a drizzle of olive oil. Roast in the oven until cooked through and serve with steamed vegetables.

Navigating dietary challenges during cancer treatment requires patience, flexibility, and creativity. By implementing these practical tips and trying out nutrient-rich recipes, you can ensure that your body receives the necessary nutrients to support your well-being and enhance your body's ability to battle cancer.

11

MOVEMENT AND EXERCISE: STRENGHTENING THE BODY, NUTURING THE SOUL

As you navigate through treatment, recovery, and survivorship, incorporating movement into your life can play a vital role in energizing the healing process. Movement not only invigorates your body but also empowers your mind, fostering a sense of strength, resilience, and well-being. In this chapter, we will explore the vitality of movement and its profound impact on the healing process.

Engaging in regular physical activity offers a multitude of benefits for cancer patients and survivors. Exercise strengthens the cardiovascular system, boosts immune function, improves muscle strength and flexibility, enhances bone density, and promotes overall physical fitness. By engaging in movement, you are providing your body with the energy it needs to heal, rebuild, and thrive.

Cardiovascular Exercise. Cardiovascular exercise, also known as aerobic exercise, is any activity that increases your heart rate and breathing. This includes brisk walking, jogging, cycling, swimming, dancing, and many other activities. Cardiovascular exercise improves the efficiency of your heart and lungs, enhances circulation, and increases oxygen delivery to your tissues. It helps to reduce fatigue, increase energy levels, and improve overall endurance.

Strength Training. Strength training exercises involve using resistance, such as weights or resistance bands, to build muscle strength and tone. Engaging in regular strength training not only helps to preserve and build lean muscle mass but also supports bone health. It can improve your ability to perform daily tasks, enhance balance and stability, and reduce the risk of falls. Strength training exercises can be adapted to your fitness level and specific needs, ensuring a safe and effective workout routine.

Flexibility and Stretching. Maintaining flexibility and joint mobility is essential for overall physical well-being. Stretching exercises help to improve flexibility, increase range of motion, and reduce muscle tension. They can alleviate stiffness, enhance posture, and promote relaxation. Incorporating stretching exercises into your routine can improve your overall physical comfort and make everyday activities easier to perform.

Mind-Body Practices. Mind-body practices, such as yoga, tai chi, and qigong, combine movement, breath control, and mindfulness to promote physical and mental well-being. These practices emphasize the connection between the mind and body, fostering a sense of harmony and balance. Mind-body exercises can help reduce stress, anxiety, and depression, while promoting relaxation, focus, and inner peace. They provide an opportunity to cultivate mindfulness and develop a deeper connection with your body.

Adapting to Individual Needs. It is essential to adapt your movement routine to your individual needs, taking into account your current fitness level, treatment regimen, and any physical limitations. Consult with your healthcare team or a qualified exercise specialist to create a personalized exercise plan that suits your abilities and goals. They can provide guidance on appropriate exercises, intensity levels, and safety precautions.

Overcoming Challenges. Embarking on a movement journey may come with challenges, such as fatigue, treatment side effects, or emotional barriers. It is crucial to listen to your body and honor its needs. Start slowly and gradually increase the intensity and duration of your exercise routine. Find activities that bring you joy and make you feel good. Seek support from loved ones, support groups, or professional counselors to address any emotional challenges that may arise. Remember, every step you take towards movement is a step towards enhancing your well-being.

The vitality of movement in the healing process cannot be overstated. Whether it is cardiovascular exercise, strength training, flexibility and stretching, or mind-body practices, each form of movement has its unique benefits. Adapt your routine to your individual needs, listen to your body, and seek support when needed. Embrace the vitality of movement, and let it be a catalyst for energizing your healing process, empowering your mind, and renewing your sense of vitality and well-being.

EXERCISE FOR CANCER RECOVERY: TAILORING PHYSICAL ACTIVITY

Physical activity plays a crucial role in the recovery process for individuals battling cancer. Exercise not only strengthens the body but also has a profound impact on the mind, enhancing overall well-being and quality of life.

Engaging in regular exercise during cancer recovery offers a wide range of benefits. It helps to counteract the side effects of treatment, such as fatigue, muscle weakness, and reduced endurance. Physical activity improves cardiovascular health, enhances immune function, and promotes weight management. It also reduces the risk of developing chronic diseases, such as heart disease and diabetes, and improves bone density.

When it comes to exercise during cancer recovery, it's essential to tailor physical activity to meet individual needs, taking into consideration factors such as the type and stage of cancer, treatment protocols, overall fitness level, and any physical limitations. It's always recommended to consult with your healthcare team before starting or modifying an exercise program.

TYPES OF EXERCISE FOR CANCER RECOVERY

1.   Cardiovascular Exercise
a.   *Walking.* Walking is a low-impact exercise that can be easily incorporated into daily routines.
b.   *Cycling.* Stationary or outdoor cycling provides an excellent cardiovascular workout while being gentle on the joints.

c. *Swimming.* Swimming and water aerobics are ideal for individuals who experience joint pain or have limited mobility.

2. Strength Training

a. *Resistance Bands.* Using resistance bands allows for a safe and effective way to build strength without placing excessive strain on the joints.

b. *Weight Training.* Gradually introducing weights can help improve muscle strength and promote bone health.

c. *Bodyweight Exercises.* Exercises such as squats, lunges, and push-ups can be done without the need for additional equipment.

3. Flexibility and Stretching

a. *Yoga.* Yoga incorporates gentle stretching, breathing exercises, and relaxation techniques, promoting flexibility, balance, and stress reduction.

b. *Pilates.* Pilates focuses on core strength, flexibility, and posture, helping to improve overall body alignment and control.

4. Mind-Body Practices

Mind-body practices, also known as mindful movement practices, are ancient practices usually composed of a combination of slow, flowing movements with deep breathing and mindfulness, aimed at promoting relaxation, balance, and coordination. They include: *Meditation, Yoga, Tai Chi,* among others. These practices help reduce stress, promote emotional well-being, and enhance overall mental clarity and focus. In the pages that follow, we will explore these techniques and how to go about them.

Safety is paramount when engaging in exercise especially during cancer recovery. It is crucial to start slowly and gradually increase the intensity and duration of physical activity. Listen to your body and rest when needed. If you experience any unusual symptoms or discomfort during exercise, consult with your healthcare team immediately. One can also consider joining support groups or exercise classes specifically designed for individuals in cancer recovery. Engage in activities that bring you joy and provide a sense of accomplishment.

Embrace the power of exercise as an essential component of your cancer recovery journey, and let it empower you to regain control of your health and thrive.

MINDFUL MOVEMENT: YOGA, TAI CHI, AND QI GONG FOR WELL-BEING

Mindful movement practices are rooted in ancient traditions that recognize the interconnectedness of the body, mind, and spirit. They emphasize the importance of nurturing both physical and emotional well-being. By engaging in these practices, individuals can experience a sense of balance, improved vitality, and a deep connection to their inner selves.

Mindful movement practices, such as yoga, Tai Chi, and Qi Gong, offer a unique approach to physical activity by combining gentle movements, breathing techniques, and a focus on present-moment awareness.

YOGA

Yoga is a practice that combines physical postures (asanas), breathing exercises (pranayama), and meditation. It offers a multitude of benefits for individuals in cancer recovery, including:

1. *Physical Well-being.* Certain yoga practices, such as inverted poses and deep breathing techniques, promote healthy blood flow and lymphatic drainage, which can support the body's natural detoxification processes.
2. *Improved flexibility.* Yoga postures gently stretch the muscles, tendons, and ligaments, promoting greater range of motion.
3. *Increased strength.* Holding yoga poses helps build strength, which is essential for maintaining overall physical function.
4. *Enhanced balance.* Balancing poses in yoga improve stability and reduce the risk of falls.

5. *Emotional Well-being.* Engaging in yoga empowers cancer patients to take an active role in their healing journey, providing a sense of control and self-efficacy. Yoga also cultivates emotional resilience by teaching patients how to stay present, manage emotions, and develop a positive mindset, helping them cope with the challenges of cancer treatment.

6. *Stress reduction.* Yoga encourages deep breathing and relaxation, leading to a reduction in stress levels.

7. *Mood enhancement.* The mindful movement and meditation aspects of yoga contribute to improved mood and emotional well-being.

8. *Self-compassion.* Yoga fosters a sense of self-acceptance and compassion, helping individuals navigate the emotional challenges of cancer recovery.

YOGA TECHNIQUES

1. *Asanas.* Asanas are physical postures designed to promote strength, flexibility, balance, and body awareness. Here are a few commonly practiced asanas:

a. Mountain Pose (Tadasana): Stand tall with feet hip-width apart, grounding through all four corners of your feet. Engage your core, lengthen your spine, and relax your shoulders. Breathe deeply and feel rooted in the present moment.

b. Cat-Cow Pose (Marjaryasana/Bitilasana): Start on all fours with hands under shoulders and knees under hips. Inhale, arch your back, and lift your chest (cow pose). Exhale, round your spine, tuck your chin, and draw your navel towards your spine (cat pose). Repeat in a flowing motion, synchronizing breath with movement.

c. Child's Pose (Balasana): Kneel on the floor, sit back on your heels, and fold your torso forward, resting your forehead on the mat. Extend your arms forward or place them alongside your body. Breathe deeply and allow your body to relax and release tension.

2. *Pranayama.* Pranayama involves conscious control and regulation of breath. These techniques can help calm the mind, increase energy, and balance the nervous system. Here are two simple pranayama techniques to try:

a. Deep Belly Breathing: Sit comfortably with a straight spine. Place one hand on your belly and the other on your chest. Inhale deeply through your nose, allowing your belly to expand, and exhale fully through your nose, letting your belly contract. Focus on the sensation of your breath moving in and out.

b. Alternate Nostril Breathing (Nadi Shodhana): Close your right nostril with your right thumb and inhale through your left nostril. Close your left nostril with your ring finger, release your right nostril, and exhale through your right nostril. Inhale through your right nostril, close it with your thumb, release your left nostril, and exhale through your left nostril. Continue this alternating pattern for several breaths.

3. *Yoga Nidra (Yogic Sleep).* Yoga Nidra is a guided relaxation technique that induces a deep state of relaxation and promotes restorative rest. Follow these steps to experience Yoga Nidra:

a. Lie down in a comfortable position, close your eyes, and bring your awareness to your breath.

b. Follow the guidance of a Yoga Nidra recording or instructor, who will lead you through a series of body scans and visualizations to help you relax each part of your body and enter a state of deep relaxation.

c. Allow yourself to fully surrender and let go, as you experience a profound sense of peace and rejuvenation.

4. *Restorative Yoga.* Restorative yoga focuses on relaxation and rejuvenation, using props such as bolsters, blankets, and blocks to support the body in gentle poses. This practice promotes deep relaxation, stress relief, and healing. Consider trying the following restorative pose:

a. Supported Bridge Pose: Lie on your back with your knees bent and feet flat on the floor. Place a bolster or folded blanket under your sacrum, supporting your lower back. Relax your arms by your sides, close your eyes, and breathe deeply. Stay in this pose for several minutes, allowing your body to surrender and release tension.

Remember, yoga is a personal journey, and it's essential to listen to your body and practice within your own limits. Start slowly and gradually increase the intensity and duration of your practice. It's also beneficial to seek guidance from a qualified yoga instructor, especially if you're new to yoga or have specific health concerns.

TAI CHI

Tai Chi is a gentle martial art characterized by slow, flowing movements and deep breathing. It focuses on cultivating a calm and meditative state of mind while promoting physical well-being. Some key benefits of Tai Chi for individuals in cancer recovery include:

1. *Balance and Coordination.* Tai Chi movements emphasize stability and weight shifting, which can enhance balance and reduce the risk of falls, especially for patients experiencing weakness or side effects from cancer treatments.

2. *Boosted Cardiovascular Health.* Tai Chi is a low-impact aerobic exercise that can improve cardiovascular fitness and circulation, supporting the cardiovascular system's functioning and overall health.

3. *Enhanced coordination.* Practicing Tai Chi helps individuals improve their body awareness and coordination.

4. *Stress Reduction.* Tai Chi promotes relaxation, deep breathing, and mindfulness, which can help reduce stress and anxiety levels, providing a sense of calm and emotional well-being.

5. *Pain Management.* Tai Chi's gentle movements and focus on body awareness can help reduce pain and discomfort associated with cancer and its treatments. It can also provide a distraction from chronic pain, promoting a sense of well-being.

6. *Improved Mood and Mental Well-Being.* Regular practice of Tai Chi has been associated with improved mood, decreased symptoms of depression, and increased overall mental well-being.

7. *Mindfulness.* Tai Chi encourages a state of mindfulness, bringing attention to the present moment and fostering a sense of calm.

TAI CHI TECHNIQUES

1. *Wu Ji Zhuang.* Wu Ji Zhang, also known as the "Wu Chi Posture" or "Standing Meditation," is a foundational practice in many Chinese internal martial arts, including Tai Chi. It is a simple yet profound stance that cultivates relaxation, body alignment, and mental focus. Here are some tips to guide you in performing this technique:

a. Stand with your feet shoulder-width apart, toes pointing forward.
b. Relax your shoulders, lengthen your spine, and tuck in your chin.
c. Allow your arms to hang naturally by your sides.
d. Distribute your weight evenly between both feet, feeling rooted and grounded.
e. Breathe deeply, directing your attention to your body and breath.
2. *Warm-up Exercises.*

a. *Neck Rolls.* Gently roll your head in a circular motion, starting from one side and moving to the other. Release any tension in your neck and shoulders.
b. *Shoulder Rolls.* Lift your shoulders towards your ears, roll them backward in a circular motion, and then relax them down.
c. *Arm Swings.* Stand with feet shoulder-width apart, extend your arms parallel to the ground, and swing them forward and backward in a relaxed manner.

d. *Leg Swings*. Stand next to a support (e.g., a chair or wall), swing one leg forward and backward in a controlled motion, and then switch to the other leg.

e. *Waist Twists*. Place your hands on your hips, gently rotate your torso from side to side, keeping your feet stable.

and intensity.

3. *Deep Diaphragmatic Breathing*. Stand or sit comfortably with a straight spine. Inhale deeply through your nose, allowing your belly to expand, and exhale fully through your mouth, letting your belly contract. Focus on slow, smooth, and relaxed breaths, allowing your body and mind to relax.

4. *Partner Work*. In advanced stages of Tai Chi practice, individuals may engage in partner work, known as Push Hands. This involves applying Tai Chi principles to engage in gentle, balanced, and cooperative pushing movements with a partner. This practice helps cultivate sensitivity, balance, and responsiveness.

It is also necessary to note that learning Tai Chi from a qualified instructor is highly recommended, especially if you're new to the practice or have specific health concerns. They can guide you in proper alignment, posture, and transitions, ensuring you receive the full benefits of Tai Chi while minimizing the risk of injury.

QI GONG

Qi Gong is an ancient Chinese practice that combines gentle movements, breath control, and meditation. It focuses on balancing the body's vital energy, known as "Qi." By incorporating Qi Gong into their cancer recovery journey, individuals can experience the following benefits:

1.   *Energy Enhancement.* Qi Gong exercises help balance and replenishment, leading to increased energy levels and reduced fatigue, a common side effect of cancer and its treatments.

2.   *Increased vitality.* Qi Gong exercises help cultivate and balance the body's energy, leading to increased vitality and well-being.

3.   *Improved Immune Function.* Regular practice of Qi Gong has been shown to enhance immune function, which is crucial for cancer patients as it supports the body's ability to fight against cancer cells and infections. It stimulates the flow of Qi (vital energy) and improves the circulation of blood and lymph, facilitating the delivery of nutrients and oxygen to cells while removing waste products.

4.   *Stress reduction.* Qi Gong helps calm the mind, reduce anxiety, and promote relaxation, which is beneficial for cancer patients who often experience high levels of stress. By focusing on slow, deliberate movements and deep breathing, Qi Gong activates the body's relaxation response, leading to a decrease in stress hormones and a sense of overall calmness.

5.   *Mind-Body Connection.* Qi Gong emphasizes the mind-body connection, helping individuals become more aware of their bodies and promoting a sense of unity between the mind, body, and spirit. Through focused attention and intention, Qi Gong cultivates mindfulness and self-awareness, facilitating a deeper understanding of one's own physical and emotional well-being.

6. *Improved focus.* Qi Gong incorporates meditation techniques that enhance mental clarity and concentration.

7. *Enhanced Physical Function.* Qi Gong exercises promote flexibility, coordination, and balance, which can be particularly beneficial for cancer patients who may experience physical limitations or side effects of treatments that affect mobility.

8. *Emotional well-being.* Regular practice of Qi Gong can help individuals manage anxiety, depression, and emotional distress associated with cancer.

9. *Pain Management.* Qi Gong exercises can help reduce pain and discomfort associated with cancer and its treatments. By improving blood and energy circulation, Qi Gong can reduce inflammation, relieve tension in the muscles and joints, and alleviate pain symptoms.

QI GONG TECHNIQUES

1. *San Yuan Zhuang (Three-Circle Standing).* The San Yuan Zhuang technique is quite connected to the Wu Ji posture earlier described. To begin this technique, assume the Wu Ji posture as described above.

a.   Visualize three circles surrounding your body at chest level, abdomen level, and hip level.

b.   Slowly rotate your upper body in a circular motion, following the path of each circle.

c.   Coordinate the movement with your breath, inhaling as you move forward and exhaling as you move backward.

d.   Feel the gentle stretching and opening of your torso, promoting relaxation and energy flow.

2. *Ba Duan Jin.* To begin with, stand with your feet shoulder-width apart, knees slightly bent, and arms relaxed by your sides. You are to perform a series of eight exercises—hence the name "Eight Pieces of Brocade"—each focusing on a specific area of the body:

a. *Two Hands Hold Up the Heavens.* Raise your arms above your head, palms facing upward, as you inhale deeply. Lower your arms as you exhale.

b. *Drawing the Bow.* Extend your left arm forward, right arm back, as if pulling a bow. Switch sides and repeat.

c. *Separating Heaven and Earth.* Interlace your fingers in front of your body, palms facing outward. Inhale, raise your arms above your head, and exhale, lower them to the sides.

d. *Wise Owl Gazes Backwards.* Turn your head to the left, looking over your shoulder, then to the right. Repeat the movement several times.

e. *Swaying the Tail.* Stand with your feet shoulder-width apart, hands resting on your lower back. Gently twist your torso from side to side, allowing your arms to swing loosely.

f. *Two Hands Support the Heavens.* Raise your arms above your head, palms facing upward, as you inhale deeply. Lower your arms as you exhale.

g. *Clenching Fists and Glaring Eyes.* Make fists with your hands and bring them close to your body, as if you are angry. Open your fists and extend your fingers, imagining releasing any tension or negativity.

h. *Bouncing on the Toes.* Rise up onto the balls of your feet, bouncing gently in place. Feel a sense of lightness and energy flowing through your body.

Perform each exercise slowly and mindfully, coordinating the movement with your breath.

3.   *Five-Element Qi Gong.* This practice focuses on connecting with the five elements of nature: wood, fire, earth, metal, and water.

To begin, stand with your feet shoulder-width apart and your arms relaxed by your sides. Visualize each element and its associated qualities while performing specific movements:

a.   *Wood.* Imagine a tall, strong tree. Extend your arms outward and sway gently from side to side, as if you are a tree in the wind.

b.   *Fire.* Picture a warm, radiant flame. Bring your hands together in front of your chest, palms facing each other, and move them apart and back together, as if you are fanning a flame.

c.   *Earth.* Envision stability and grounding. Place your hands on your lower abdomen and gently rotate your hips in a circular motion.

d.   *Metal.* Visualize purity and strength. Bring your arms up in front of your chest, palms facing downward, and press downward, as if you are molding metal.

e.   *Water.* Imagine flowing, adaptable energy. Extend your arms outward and move them in a wave-like motion, as if you are swimming through water.

4.   *Dan Tian Breathing.*

a.   Sit or stand in a comfortable position, with your spine straight and your shoulders relaxed.

b.   Place one hand on your lower abdomen, just below your navel, and the other hand on your chest.

c.   Breathe deeply into your lower abdomen, feeling it expand as you inhale. Allow your chest to rise slightly.

d.   Exhale slowly and completely, feeling your abdomen contract and your chest sink.

e.   Focus your attention on the breath, allowing it to become deep, smooth, and rhythmic.

Conclusion:

Qi Gong offers a holistic approach to cultivating vital energy and inner harmony. By practicing these techniques regularly, you can experience a multitude of benefits, including reduced stress, improved relaxation, enhanced physical and mental well-being, increased energy, improved balance and coordination, and a greater sense of overall harmony. Remember to approach the practice with patience, curiosity, and an open heart. Embrace the journey of Qi Gong as a pathway to self-discovery and self-care, supporting your well-being on all levels – body, mind, and spirit

Mindful movement practices offer a holistic approach to physical activity and well-being during the cancer recovery process. Integrating these practices into your daily routine can be a transformative experience. Start by finding a qualified instructor who specializes in working with individuals in cancer recovery. They can guide you through appropriate modifications and provide personalized support. Begin with gentle and beginner-friendly classes and gradually progress at your own pace. Remember, the focus is on self-care, not competition or perfection. Let these ancient practices guide you on a path of healing and empowerment as you navigate the journey of cancer recovery.

PART IV

Thriving Beyond Cancer

12

REDEFINIG SUCCESS: REIMAGINING LIFE AFTER CANCER

The cancer journey is a life-altering experience that challenges us. Throughout the journey of battling cancer, individuals face numerous trials and tribulations, but with proper guidance they can also discover remarkable resilience and strength within themselves. As part of the healing process, it becomes essential to redefine success and reimagine life after cancer.

In a society often driven by external achievements and material pursuits, the concept of success can become narrow and limited. However, cancer has a unique way of shifting our perspective, prompting us to reevaluate what truly matters in life. Success, in the context of cancer recovery, is not solely defined by conventional measures such as wealth, status, or career accomplishments. It goes beyond that as it encompasses personal growth, emotional well-being, and the ability to find joy and meaning in each moment.

Striving through the journey (and eventually surviving cancer) marks the beginning of a new chapter, one that offers the opportunity for profound transformation and a fresh outlook on life. Reimagining life after cancer involves embracing the lessons learned through the battle, cultivating a sense of purpose, and nurturing a fulfilling existence. It is about finding a new balance, rediscovering passions, and fostering meaningful connections with others.

One of the fundamental aspects of redefining success and reimagining life after cancer is a shift in perspective. This shift involves letting go of societal expectations and embracing a more authentic and personally meaningful definition of success. It requires acknowledging and celebrating the strength, courage, and resilience that were developed throughout the cancer journey.

Finding fulfillment in the struggle and even after cancer is another fundamental aspect of the cancer journey. It involves reconnecting with our passions, pursuing activities that bring us joy and a sense of purpose, and cultivating meaningful relationships. It may mean exploring new hobbies, engaging in creative endeavors, or contributing to the well-being of others through volunteer work or advocacy. By aligning our lives with our values and passions, we create a sense of fulfillment that extends far beyond the confines of cancer.

Cancer can, and should, be viewed as a catalyst for personal growth and transformation. It allows us to redefine our identity beyond being a cancer patient and teaches us the profound lessons of resilience, gratitude, and the strength of the human spirit, which are crucial in envisioning a future filled with joy, purpose, and fulfillment. Through the journey, with proper guidance, we develop an unwavering belief in our ability to overcome challenges and thrive in the face of adversity. This newfound resilience becomes an essential asset as we aim at redefining success and reimagining life after cancer. By shifting our focus from external achievements to internal growth and well-being, we open ourselves up to a world of possibilities and find renewed purpose and joy and thus embrace the extraordinary possibilities that lie ahead.

SETTING NEW GOALS AND DREAMS: EMBRACING A FRESH START

Setting goals is an integral part of the healing process. Goals provide direction, motivation, and a sense of purpose. They give us something to strive for and help us focus our energy and efforts towards positive outcomes. It enables us to shift our mindset from a state of illness to one of empowerment and growth.

When setting new goals, it is crucial to ensure they are both realistic and meaningful to us. Realistic goals are attainable and take into consideration our current physical abilities, emotional state, and resources. They are goals that we can work towards with dedication and persistence. Meaningful goals, on the other hand, align with our values, passions, and aspirations. They reflect what truly matters to us and inspire us to take action.

As we work towards our goals, it is important to celebrate milestones and acknowledge the progress we have made. Each step forward, no matter how small, is a testament to our strength and resilience. Also note that setting new goals and dreams does not mean that challenges will cease to exist. It is important to acknowledge and prepare for the obstacles that may arise along the way. These challenges may be physical, emotional, or logistical in nature. Thus, by recognizing and celebrating our achievements, we fuel our motivation, boost our self-confidence, and reinforce our belief in our ability to create positive change in our lives.

EMBODYING RESILIENCE: CULTIVATING ADAPTABILITY AND INNER STRENGTH

Resilience is the ability to bounce back, adapt, and thrive in the midst of challenges. It is not about avoiding or denying the difficulties we encounter, but rather about developing the inner strength and flexibility to navigate them.

Resilience is not an innate trait but rather a skill that can be learned and developed. It is the capacity to maintain a positive outlook, persevere through difficulties, and recover from setbacks. Resilience is not about being invincible or unaffected by adversity, but rather about our ability to bounce back, grow, and learn from the experience. By cultivating resilience, we can navigate the challenges of cancer with greater ease and embrace the potential for personal growth and transformation.

Cultivating Inner Strength. Building inner strength is at the core of resilience. It involves developing a strong sense of self-belief, confidence, and self-compassion. Inner strength allows us to tap into our inner resources and draw upon our resilience during challenging times. It empowers us to face adversity with courage and determination, knowing that we have the strength within us to overcome obstacles.

Adapting to Change. Cancer diagnosis brings about significant changes in our lives, both physically and emotionally. Adapting to these changes requires flexibility and a willingness to embrace new circumstances. It involves letting go of the past and finding ways to adjust and thrive in the present. Adapting to change allows us to find new strategies, redefine our priorities, and discover alternative paths towards well-being and recovery.

Positive Mindset and Optimism. Maintaining a positive mindset and optimism are crucial aspects of cultivating resilience. A positive mindset does not mean denying the challenges or pretending that everything is perfect. It means focusing on the possibilities, finding silver linings, and maintaining hope in the face of adversity. By adopting an optimistic outlook, we can reframe difficulties as opportunities for growth and embrace a sense of possibility and empowerment.

Developing Coping Strategies. Coping strategies are tools and techniques that help us navigate the emotional and physical challenges of cancer. These strategies can vary from person to person and may include relaxation techniques, mindfulness practices, seeking social support, engaging in creative outlets, or participating in support groups. By developing and implementing effective coping strategies, we can manage stress, reduce anxiety, and enhance our overall well-being.

Building Supportive Relationships. The presence of a supportive network is invaluable in cultivating resilience. Surrounding ourselves with caring and understanding individuals can provide emotional support, encouragement, and practical assistance. Building and nurturing relationships with loved ones, friends, and support groups create a sense of belonging and connectedness, which strengthens our resilience during difficult times

Embracing Self-Care. Self-care is an essential component of resilience. It involves prioritizing our physical, emotional, and mental well-being. Engaging in activities that bring us joy, practicing self-compassion, and prioritizing rest and relaxation are crucial for maintaining resilience. By caring for ourselves, we replenish our energy, enhance our ability to cope with challenges, and promote our overall health and well-being.

Learning and Growth. Resilience is a dynamic process that involves continuous learning and growth. Each experience, setback, and triumph can serve as a catalyst for personal development. By embracing a growth mindset and viewing challenges as opportunities for learning, we can transform adversity into resilience, strength, and wisdom. Learning from our experiences allows us to build resilience for future challenges and navigate the cancer journey with greater adaptability and inner strength.

Embodying resilience is a transformative journey that empowers us to navigate the challenges of a cancer diagnosis with adaptability, inner strength, and optimism and thrive amidst the adversities we face.

CELEBRATING MILESTONES: EMBRACING LIFE'S VICTORIES ALONG THE WAY

In the journey of battling cancer, it is essential to recognize and celebrate the milestones that we achieve along the way. Embracing life's victories along the cancer journey is a powerful act of self-empowerment and resilience. Each step forward, each victory, no matter how small, is a testament to our resilience, strength, and determination. It is about recognizing and celebrating our progress, finding meaning and purpose, practicing gratitude and appreciation, engaging in self-reflection and growth, creating meaningful rituals, and inspiring others through our stories. Each milestone we celebrate becomes a testament to our strength, a reminder of our capacity to overcome challenges, and a source of hope for the future.

Acknowledging progress is about recognizing and celebrating the small steps we take towards healing and recovery. It is easy to become focused on the end goal of being cancer-free, but it is equally important to celebrate the incremental improvements we make along the way. Whether it is completing a round of chemotherapy, reaching a new level of physical strength, or experiencing a moment of emotional breakthrough, each milestone is a cause for celebration.

Creating rituals and ceremonies around milestones can provide a sense of significance and mark important moments in our cancer journey. These rituals can be as simple as lighting a candle, writing in a journal, or gathering with loved ones to commemorate a particular milestone. By creating these rituals, we honor our achievements, express gratitude, and foster a sense of community and support.

Self-reflection is another essential aspect of celebrating milestones. It involves taking the time to reflect on our journey, the lessons learned, and the personal growth that has occurred. By pausing and reflecting on our experiences, we gain valuable insights into our strengths, resilience, and areas of personal development. Each milestone becomes an opportunity for self-reflection and a reminder of the progress we have made.

Sharing our milestones and victories with others can have a profound impact, not only on ourselves but also on those around us. By sharing our stories, we can inspire hope and resilience in others who may be going through similar experiences. Celebrating our milestones becomes an opportunity to uplift and support others on their own cancer journey. It reminds us that we are not alone and that our experiences can make a positive difference in the lives of others.

13

PAYING IT FORWARD: SHAPING YOUR JOURNEY TO INSPIRE OTHERS

There arises a very powerful opportunity in the journey of battling cancer—a chance to pay it forward and share your journey to inspire others. When we face adversity and navigate the challenges of illness, we gain valuable insights, strength, and resilience that can serve as a guiding light for those who may be walking a similar path.

When we share our cancer journey, we create a ripple effect that extends far beyond ourselves. Our experiences, emotions, and lessons learned have the power to touch the lives of others, offering hope, encouragement, and guidance. By sharing the ups and downs, the triumphs and setbacks, we build a sense of connection and community. Through our vulnerability and authenticity, we show others that they are not alone and that it is possible to find strength and resilience in the face of adversity.

Sharing your cancer journey is an act of inspiring hope and resilience. By sharing your story, you offer a ray of light to those who may be feeling lost or overwhelmed. Your journey becomes a source of inspiration, reminding others that they too have the inner strength to face their challenges head-on. Through your experiences, you provide a roadmap for navigating the twists and turns of the cancer journey, offering insights, strategies, and a glimpse of what is possible.

When you share your cancer journey, you create a space for connection and support. Others who have gone through or are currently facing similar battles can relate to your experiences and find solace in knowing that they are not alone. By sharing your highs and lows, you foster a sense of camaraderie and empathy. Through this shared connection, you become a pillar of support, offering encouragement, understanding, and a listening ear.

Sharing your journey also empowers others to speak up and share their own stories. Often, individuals may feel hesitant or uncertain about sharing their struggles, fearing judgment or misunderstanding. By courageously opening up about your experiences, you create a safe and accepting space for others to do the same. You give them permission to voice their fears, hopes, and dreams. Through this empowerment, you contribute to breaking the silence and reducing the stigma surrounding cancer.

You also contribute to spreading awareness and education about the disease by sharing your experience. Your firsthand account offers a unique perspective that textbooks and statistics cannot provide. By sharing information about the symptoms, treatments, and resources you have encountered, you empower others to become informed advocates for their own health. Through education, you become an agent of change, ensuring that others are equipped with the knowledge they need to make informed decisions and seek appropriate support.

By sharing your journey, one tends to leave a lasting legacy. Your experiences, wisdom, and resilience become part of a collective tapestry of hope and inspiration. Your story lives on in the hearts and minds of those you touch, continuing to uplift and empower them even after you have moved beyond the challenges of cancer. By paying it forward and sharing your journey, you create a positive impact that extends far into the future.

Paying it forward by sharing your cancer journey is a profound act of courage, compassion, and empowerment. It inspires hope, fosters connection, and spreads awareness. Embrace the opportunity to pay it forward and let your light shine brightly for others to see and be inspired by.

FINDING YOUR VOICE: SHARING YOUR CANCER EXPERIENCE WITH AUTHENTICITY

When faced with a cancer diagnosis, one of the most powerful tools at our disposal is our own voice. Sharing our cancer experience with authenticity allows us to express our thoughts, emotions, and fears, while also providing a source of inspiration and support for others. In finding our voice, we give ourselves permission to be vulnerable and create connections that can enhance our healing journey.

Authenticity is the 'key' when sharing our cancer experience. It means being true to ourselves and expressing our thoughts and emotions without filters or masks. By sharing our authentic selves, we invite others to connect with us on a deeper level, creating a space where empathy and understanding can flourish. It is through this authenticity that we find strength and resilience.

Sharing our cancer experience with authenticity also allows us to reclaim our narrative. Rather than allowing cancer to define us, we take ownership of our story and become the authors of our lives. In doing so, we empower ourselves and inspire others to do the same. Our journey becomes a testament to the power of the human spirit and the ability to rise above adversity.

As we navigate the challenges of cancer, we have the opportunity to become advocates for ourselves and others. We become a voice for those who may not have the strength or platform to speak out. Being an advocate means standing up for what we believe in and working to effect positive change. It involves educating ourselves about the disease, treatment options, and support resources available. Armed with knowledge, we can empower ourselves and others to make informed decisions and take control of our health.

Advocacy also extends beyond raising awareness. It involves supporting and uplifting others who are on their own cancer journey. By offering a listening ear, sharing resources, and providing encouragement, we become a source of strength for those in need. Summarily, advocacy is all about creating a community of support where no one feels alone in their battle.

In the spirit of authentic living, we leave a lasting legacy behind that, even without our knowledge, serve as a source of inspiration and courage to others. Leaving a legacy involves using our experiences to create positive change and inspire others long after we are gone. It is about leaving behind a footprint of hope and resilience.

One way to leave a legacy is by sharing our stories through various mediums. Whether it's writing a book, creating art, or speaking at events, our stories have the power to touch and inspire others. By sharing our wisdom and lessons learned, we provide guidance and comfort to those who follow in our footsteps.

Leaving a legacy also involves giving back to the community. It may be through volunteering, supporting cancer research initiatives, or starting a foundation. It can also be as simple as providing support and assistance in social media groups or platforms. By contributing our time, resources, and expertise, we ensure that our impact extends beyond our own journey and into the lives of others.

Ultimately, the power of authenticity, becoming an advocate, and leaving a legacy lies in the ripple effect it creates. Each person we touch, each life we inspire, has the potential to pass on the torch of hope and resilience to others. Together, we can build a community that supports and uplifts each other in the face of adversity.

In the face of cancer, we become a force for change, our advocacy becomes a source of strength, and our legacies become beacons of hope. It is through these actions that we not only navigate our own journey but also light the way for others, reminding them that they are not alone. Together, we can harness the power of the mind, find healing, and create a world where cancer is overcome with resilience, determination, and unwavering hope

CONCLUSION: LIVING WITH PURPOSE AND GRATITUDE

In the journey of battling cancer, one of the most profound transformations we can experience is the awakening of living with purpose and gratitude. It is in these moments of reflection and introspection that we realize the true value of each precious day and the immense power of our own minds.

Living with purpose means embracing each day as a gift and finding meaning in even the smallest of moments. It is about setting intentions and aligning our actions with our values. In the face of adversity, we discover a newfound clarity and determination to make a positive impact in the world. We become inspired to pursue our dreams, to mend broken relationships, and to live authentically, guided by a deep understanding of what truly matters in life.

Gratitude becomes a guiding light, illuminating the beauty that surrounds us amidst the challenges. It is a transformative practice that shifts our perspective, allowing us to see the blessings that often go unnoticed. In the face of cancer, we learn to appreciate the simplest joys, the support of loved ones, and the resilience of our own spirits. Gratitude becomes a beacon of hope that sustains us, reminding us of the abundance of love, strength, and courage that resides within.

Living with purpose and gratitude intertwines the power of the mind with the depth of the soul. It is a harmonious dance between mindfulness and intentionality, where we embrace the present moment with a deep sense of gratitude while staying focused on our purpose and goals. It is through this synergy that we unlock the true potential within ourselves, transcending the limitations imposed by cancer.

As we embark on this journey, we realize that our experiences have the power to touch the lives of others. Our stories, our triumphs, and even our moments of vulnerability become beacons of inspiration for those who are walking a similar path. By living with purpose and gratitude, we become beacons of hope, radiating a light that guides others through their own battles.

In the end, the journey is not just about surviving cancer; it is about thriving in the face of adversity. It is about embracing the power of the mind, nurturing the soul, and creating a life that is deeply fulfilling. It is about cherishing every moment, cultivating meaningful connections, and leaving a legacy of love and resilience.

May this journey empower you to live with purpose, to embrace gratitude, and to discover the extraordinary strength that resides within. Let us stand together, united by the power of the mind, the resilience of the human spirit, and the unwavering belief that a life filled with purpose and gratitude is a life truly well-lived.

APPENDIX: ADDITIONAL RESOURCES FOR SUPPORT

It is essential to have access to a wide range of resources and support systems. This appendix provides a comprehensive list of additional resources that can be of help in your journey, provide valuable information, and connect you with communities dedicated to supporting individuals on their cancer journey. Explore these resources to find the support you need and empower yourself with knowledge and inspiration.

1. *Cancer Support Organizations.*
   a. American Cancer Society, www.cancer.org
   b. Cancer Research UK, www.cancerresearchuk.org
   c. Canadian Cancer Society, www.cancer.ca
   d. Australian Cancer Council, www.cancer.org.au
   e. National Cancer Institute, www.cancer.gov
   f. CancerCare, www.cancercare.org
   g. Cancer.Net, www.cancer.net
   h. OncoLink, www.oncolink.org
   i. Cancer Association of Zimbabwe, www.cancerassociationofzimbabwe.org.zw – Zimbabwe
   j. Pink Ribbon Red Ribbon, www.pinkribbonredribbon.org – Focused on cervical and breast cancer in Sub-Saharan Africa
   k. Breast Care International, www.breastcareinternational.org – Ghana
   l. Cancer Association of Namibia, www.cancernamibia.com
   m. Cancer Support Network of Zimbabwe, www.cancersupport.co.zw – Zimbabwe
   n. The Leukemia & Lymphoma Society, www.lls.org
   o. Livestrong Foundation, www.livestrong.org

p.   Susan G. Komen, www.komen.org

2.   *International Cancer Associations and Networks.*
a.   Union for International Cancer Control, www.uicc.org
b.   European Society for Medical Oncology, www.esmo.org
c.   International Association for the Study of Lung Cancer, www.iaslc.org
d.   Asia Pacific Society of Clinical Oncology, www.apsoc2020.org
e.   Latin American and Caribbean Society of Medical Oncology, www.slacom.org
f.   Cancer Association of South Africa, www.cansa.org.za
g.   Kenya Cancer Association, www.kenyacancer.org
h.   Uganda Cancer Institute, www.uci.or.ug
i.   Nigeria Cancer Society, www.nigeriacancersociety.org
j.   African Cancer Registry Network, www.afcrn.org
k.   African Organisation for Research and Training in Cancer, www.aortic-africa.org
l.   West African College of S www.wacscoac.org
m.   Pan African Association of Surgeons, www.paasurg.org

3.   *Global Cancer Research and Treatment Centers.*
a.   Cancer Research and Support Foundation, www.cancerresearchandsupport.org
b.   Memorial Sloan Kettering Cancer Center, www.mskcc.org – United States
c.   MD Anderson Cancer Center, www.mdanderson.org – United States
d.   Royal Marsden Hospital, www.royalmarsden.nhs.uk – United Kingdom

e. Peter MacCallum Cancer Centre, www.petermac.org – Australia

f. Institut Gustave Roussy, www.gustaveroussy.fr – France

g. Cancer Research Initiative Kenya, www.cri.or.ke – Kenya

h. Institute of Human Virology Nigeria, www.ihvnigeria.org

i. Makerere University College of Health Sciences, www.mak.ac.ug

j. University of Cape Town Cancer Research Initiative, www.cancer.uct.ac.za

k. American Institute for Cancer Research, www.aicr.org

l. Cancer Council Australia Nutrition, www.cancercouncil.com.au

m. World Cancer Research Fund, www.wcrf.org

n. Canadian Cancer Society Nutrition, www.cancer.ca

o. Chris Hani Baragwanath Academic Hospital, www.chrishanibaragwanathhospital.co.za – South Africa

p. Cairo University Hospitals, www.cairo-university.org – Egypt

q. Institut Jules Bordet, www.bordet.be – Belgium (also provides support to African countries)

r. African Organisation for Research and Training in Cancer, www.aortic-africa.org

s. National Cancer Institute of Egypt, www.nci.cu.edu.eg – Egypt

t. Ocean Road Cancer Institute, www.orci.or.tz – Tanzania

u. University of Ghana School of Medicine and Dentistry, www.ug.edu.gh – Ghana

v. University of Nairobi – Institute of Tropical and Infectious Diseases, www.uonbi.ac.ke

w. Stellenbosch University – Division of Medical Oncology, www.sun.ac.za

4. *Physical Activity and Exercise Resources.*
a. American College of Sports Medicine, www.acsm.org
b. Exercise & Sports Science Australia, www.essa.org.au
c. Canadian Society for Exercise Physiology, www.csep.ca
d. European Society of Sports Traumatology, Knee Surgery and Arthroscopy, www.esska.org

5. *Financial Assistance and Support.*
a. Cancer Financial Assistance Coalition, www.cancerfac.org
b. CancerCare Financial Assistance, www.cancercare.org
c. Cancer Council Australia Financial Assistance, www.cancer.org.au
d. Macmillan Cancer Support Financial Help, www.macmillan.org.uk
e. Cancer Association of South Africa, www.cansa.org.za
f. Kenya Cancer Association, www.kenyacancer.org
g. Uganda Cancer Society, www.ugandacancersociety.org
h. Cancer Association of South Africa, www.cansa.org.za
i. Ghana Cancer Registry, www.ghanahealthservice.org/cancer
j. Cancer Association of Botswana, www.cancerassociationofbotswana.com

6. *Palliative Care and Hospice Services.*
a. Worldwide Hospice Palliative Care Alliance, www.thewhpca.org
b. Hospice Foundation of America, www.hospicefoundation.org
c. European Association for Palliative Care, www.eapcnet.eu

d. Australian and New Zealand Society of Palliative Medicine, www.anzspm.org.au
e. African Palliative Care Association, www.africanpalliativecare.org
f. Hospice Africa Uganda, www.hospiceafrica.or.ug
g. Hospice Kenya, www.hospicecarekenya.com
h. Hospice and Palliative Care Association of South Africa, www.hpca.co.za

7. *Mind-Body Medicine Resources.*
a. The Chopra Center, www.chopra.com
b. The Center for Mind-Body Medicine, www.cmbm.org
c. The Benson-Henry Institute for Mind Body Medicine, www.bensonhenryinstitute.org
d. The Healing Mind, www.thehealingmind.org

8. *Meditation and Mindfulness Apps.*
a. Headspace, www.headspace.com
b. Calm, www.calm.com
c. Insight Timer, www.insighttimer.com
d. Aura, www.aurahealth.io
e. Stop, Breathe & Think, www.stopbreathethink.com

9. *Online Support Communities.*
a. Cancer Survivors Network, csn.cancer.org
b. Inspire, www.inspire.com
c. Smart Patients, www.smartpatients.com
d. Cancer Support Community, www.cancersupportcommunity.org
e. Macmillan Cancer Support, www.macmillan.org.uk

f. Cancer Research UK Online Community,
    www.cancerresearchuk.org/about-cancer/cancer-chat

g. Cancer Council Australia Online Community,
    www.cancercouncil.com.au/forums

10. *Professional Support and Supportive Therapies.*

a. Psychologists and counselors specialized in oncology and
    mindfulness-based therapies.

b. Support groups facilitated by mental health professionals
    or cancer centers.

c. Integrative medicine practitioners who can provide
    guidance on holistic approaches to support your journey.

d. *Art therapy.* Engaging in creative expression to promote
    emotional well-being and self-discovery.

e. *Music therapy.* Utilizing music to reduce stress, enhance
    mood, and provide a sense of comfort.

f. *Yoga therapy.* Combining movement, breathwork, and
    meditation to promote physical and emotional healing.

Remember, you are not alone in your battle against cancer.
These resources can provide valuable information, emotional
support, and inspiration as you navigate your path to healing.
Explore what resonates with you and trust your intuition in
finding the resources that best suit your needs. Reach out to
these organizations, communities, and professionals, and let
their knowledge and support help guide you on your
transformative journey of healing and empowerment.

Please note that this is not an exhaustive list, and new
resources are constantly emerging. Also note that availability
and access to specific resources may vary by location. It is
important to research and seek resources specific to your

country or region to ensure the most relevant and up-to-date information and support. Be open to exploring various avenues and finding what resonates with you personally. Your journey is unique, and by embracing these additional resources, you can tap into the collective power of support and knowledge to enhance your well-being and make your journey through cancer more manageable.